Key Questions in Preventative Farm Animal Medicine

Volume 1

Types, Causes and Treatment of Infectious Diseases

Key Questions in Preventative Farm Animal Medicine

Volume 1
**Types, Causes and Treatment
of Infectious Diseases**

Edited by Tanmoy Rana

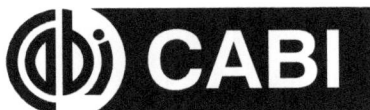

⟨ⓑ⟩ CABI

CABI is a trading name of CAB International

CABI	CABI
Nosworthy Way	200 Portland Street
Wallingford	Boston
Oxfordshire OX10 8DE	MA 02114
UK	USA

Tel: +44 (0)1491 832111
E-mail: info@cabi.org
Website: www.cabi.org

Tel: +1 (617)682-9015
E-mail: cabi-nao@cabi.org

The views expressed in this publication are those of the author(s) and do not necessarily represent those of, and should not be attributed to, CAB International (CABI). Any images, figures and tables not otherwise attributed are the author(s)' own. References to internet websites (URLs) were accurate at the time of writing.

CAB International and, where different, the copyright owner shall not be liable for technical or other errors or omissions contained herein. The information is supplied without obligation and on the understanding that any person who acts upon it, or otherwise changes their position in reliance thereon, does so entirely at their own risk. Information supplied is neither intended nor implied to be a substitute for professional advice. The reader/user accepts all risks and responsibility for losses, damages, costs and other consequences resulting directly or indirectly from using this information.

CABI's Terms and Conditions, including its full disclaimer, may be found at https://www.cabi.org/terms-and-conditions/.

A catalogue record for this book is available from the British Library, London, UK.

ISBN-13: 9781800624702 (paperback)
         9781800624719 (ePDF)
         9781800624726 (ePub)

DOI: 10.1079/9781800624726.0000

Commissioning Editor: Alexandra Lainsbury
Editorial Assistant: Emma McCann
Production Editor: James Bishop

Typeset by Straive, Pondicherry, India

Contents

Contributors   vii

Preface   ix

Acknowledgements   ix

Notes for users   x

1   **General Aspects of Preventive
    Veterinary Medicine**   1
    *Abrar Ul Haq, Biswa Ranjan Jena, Aishwarya
    Dash and Tanmoy Rana*

    Introduction   1
    Multiple Choice Questions   3
    Answers   43

2   **Viral Diseases**   45
    J.B. Kathiriya and Chetan Chavda

    Introduction   45
    Multiple Choice Questions   47
    Answers   85

3   **Bacterial Diseases**   87
    J.B. Kathiriya

    Introduction   87
    Multiple Choice Questions   89
    Answers   135

4   **Fungal Diseases**   137
    J. Jyothi and M. Bhavya Sree

    Introduction   137
    Multiple Choice Questions   139
    Answers   185

5   Mycoplasma Diseases   **187**
J.B. Kathiriya

Introduction   187
Multiple Choice Questions   189
Answers   211

6   Ectoparasitic Infestation   **212**
H. Dhanalakshmi

Introduction   212
Multiple Choice Questions   213
Answers   253

7   Endoparasitic Infections   **255**
Bhupamani Das and Sivajothi Srigireddy

Introduction   255
Multiple Choice Questions   257
Answers   297

Contributors

Chetan D. Chavda, Department of Veterinary Microbiology, College of Veterinary Science and AH, Kamdhenu University, Junagadh, Gujarat, India.

Bhupamani Das, College of Veterinary Science & AH, KU, Sardarkrushinagar, Gujarat-385506, India.

Aishwarya Dash, Division of Animal Genetics and Breeding, National Dairy Research Institute, Karnal, Haryana, India.

H. Dhanalakshmi, Department of Parasitology, Veterinary College, Hebbal, India.

Abrar Ul Haq, Department of Veterinary Medicine, Guru Angad Dev Veterinary and Animal Sciences University, Ludhiana, Punjab, India.

Biswa Ranjan Jena, Department of Veterinary Medicine, Guru Angad Dev Veterinary and Animal Sciences University, Ludhiana, Punjab, India.

J. Jyothi, Department of Veterinary Medicine, P.V. Narasimharao Telangana Veterinary University, Hyderabad, India.

J.B. Kathiriya, Department of Veterinary Microbiology, College of Veterinary Science and AH, Kamdhenu University, Junagadh, Gujarat, India; Department of Veterinary Public Health, Kamdhenu University, Junagadh, India.

Tanmoy Rana, Department of Veterinary Clinical Complex, F/VAS, WBUAFS, Kolkata, India.

M. Bhavya Sree, P.V. Narasimharao Telangana Veterinary University, Hyderabad, India.

Sivajothi Srigireddy, College of Veterinary Science, Proddatur, Andhrapradesh-516360, India.

Preface

This book consists solely of multiple choice questions (MCQs), designed for anyone engaged in the study of veterinary science, in particular those aiming to take examinations such as national eligibility tests, DVM/BVSc and AH examinations, postgraduate study and junior and senior research fellowships. There are seven chapters, dealing with all aspects of farm animal medicine, compiled by a range of experienced authors, based on the most up-to-date knowledge in the field, and each including a brief introduction. The questions are analytical and comprehensive in nature and should be used alongside students' wider reading around their subject and their classroom learning.

Acknowledgements

I would like to convey my sincere gratitude to the Honourable Vice Chancellor, West Bengal University of Animal & Fishery Sciences, Kolkata, India, for providing me with the opportunity to edit this series of MCQ books. I am grateful to all contributors who wholeheartedly helped me by providing their chapters so swiftly. I am also indebted to my colleagues for useful advice. I am thankful to all the personnel at CAB International for providing me with the opportunity to act as editor for this series. I would also like to thank my family for providing great support and the time to finalize each book.

Tanmoy Rana
Kolkata, India

Notes for users

The use of MCQs is common in formative and summative examination. MCQs are composed of one question (stem) with four possible answers, including the correct answer and several incorrect answers (distractors). One correct answer must be selected from the four possible responses to the stem.

1

General Aspects of Preventive Veterinary Medicine

Abrar Ul Haq, Biswa Ranjan Jena, Aishwarya Dash and Tanmoy Rana

Introduction

Infectious diseases of farm animals are one of the major threats to agriculture and can cause considerable damage at local, regional and even international levels, both in industrialized and in developing countries. For example, the production of calves in a cattle farm can be seriously affected by virus- or bacteria-induced abortions. Diseases of domestic animals not only affect animal production and animal trade but can, in some cases, be transmitted and cause diseases in humans (zoonoses). In some cases the economy of a whole country can be threatened by animal pathogens that have a direct effect on production efficiency, but also have various indirect effects on the international trade of animals and animal-derived products. In the last two centuries, considerable efforts have been invested in understanding the causes and pathogenesis of viral and bacterial diseases in domestic animals. These studies have introduced new methodologies for the diagnosis, treatment and control of veterinary diseases. Importantly, research on veterinary pathogens has also had a major impact on understanding the basic biological processes of viruses and bacteria. In some cases, studies of veterinary pathogens have revolutionized biology and established entire new disciplines. The questions in this chapter take a general perspective on those farm animal diseases – bacterial, viral, parasitic, protozoal, fungal and rickettsial – that have made a major contribution to the current understanding of pathogen biology.

These questions concern the most common and important infectious diseases prevalent in farm animals like cattle, buffalo, sheep, goats, pigs and horses. They cover the aetiology, diagnosis, treatment, prevention and control of diseases such as anthrax, BQ, HS, FMD, MCF, rabies, mastitis, babesiosis, theileriosis, bluetongue, PPR, Johne's disease, glanders, strangles, classical swine fever, African swine fever, equine infectious anaemia, EHV, tetanus and dermatophytosis among many others.

© CAB International 2024. *Key Questions in Preventative Farm Animal Medicine*
Volume 1: Types, Causes and Treatment of Infectious Diseases (ed. T. Rana)
DOI: 10.1079/9781800624726.0001

Multiple Choice Questions

1. **In neonates, the most common form of *E. coli* reported in outbreaks of enteritis is:**

   a. Enterotoxic

   b. Enterohemorrhagic

   c. Necrotoxic

   d. Verotoxic

2. **Enzootic abortion in sheep is seen in:**

   a. Brucellosis

   b. Chlamydiosis

   c. Campylobacteriosis

   d. All of these

3. **Louping-ill in sheep is characterized by:**

   a. Meningitis

   b. Encephalitis

   c. Bouncing gait

   d. All of these

4. **Empyema of the guttural pouch in horses is a complication of:**

   a. Glanders

   b. Strangles

   c. Botryomycosis

   d. Histoplasmosis

5. **Pink eye in cattle is caused by:**

   a. *Streptococcus pneumoniae*

   b. *Staphylococcus aureus*

   c. *Moraxella bovis*

   d. *Dermatophilus congolensis*

6. **Lumpy wool in sheep is caused by:**

   a. *Fusobacterium necrophorum*

   b. *Dermatophilus congolensis*

   c. *Corynebacterium renale*

   d. *Cryptococcus neoformans*

7. **Which of the following is characteristic chlamydiosis?**

   a. Guarneir bodies

   b. Negri bodies

   c. Elementary bodies

   d. Borrel bodies

8. **Primary vaccination of FMD in calves is performed at which age?**

   a. 3 months

   b. 4 months

   c. 5 months

   d. 6 months

9. **Rigor mortis is absent in animals that have died of anthrax due to the release of:**

   a. Lethal factor

   b. Oedema factor

   c. Protective antigen

   d. All of these

10. **Sterne spore vaccine is administered against:**

    a. Brucellosis

    b. Chlamydiosis

    c. Anthrax

    d. Black quarter

11. **In mastitis, an electrical conductivity test is based on the increase in the concentration of:**

   a. Calcium ion

   b. Magnesium ion

   c. Chloride ion

   d. None of these

12. **The Californian mastitis test detects changes in what?**

   a. pH

   b. Ions

   c. Leucocytes

   d. a and c

13. **Udder impetigo in cattle is caused by:**

   a. *Staphylococcus aureus*

   b. *Streptococcus agalactiae*

   c. *Streptococcus dysgalactiae*

   d. b and c

14. **The somatic cell count (lakhs) in healthy cattle milk should be:**

   a. < 1,00,000

   b. 1,00,000–2,00,000

   c. 2,00,000–5,00,000

   d. 5,00,000–10,00,000

15. **The total number of bluetongue virus serotypes is:**

   a. 10

   b. 15

   c. 20

   d. 24

16. **Bluetongue virus affects:**

   a. Gustatory papillae

   b. Oro-pharyngeal epithelium

5

c. Vascular endothelium

d. Large intestine

17. **Erosions at the tip of the cheek papillae at the commissure of the mouth in sheep is a characteristic of:**

a. PPR

b. Contagious ecthyma

c. Vesicular stomatitis

d. FMD

18. **The wheelbarrow test is used for the diagnosis of:**

a. Ovine pulmonary adenomatosis

b. PPR

c. Listeriosis

d. Louping ill

19. **Which vaccines are used for the control of sheep and goat pox?**

a. Killed

b. Live attenuated

c. Recombinant DNA

d. Toxoid

20. **The condition big knee is seen in goats affected with:**

a. Brucellosis

b. Caprine arthritis encephalitis

c. Caseous lymphadenitis

d. None of these

21. **Transmissible gastroenteritis in pigs is caused by:**

a. Parvo virus

b. Corona virus

c. Pesti virus

d. a and b

22. **Which of the following is a fungal disease?**

    a. Epizootic lymphangitis

    b. Ulcerative lymphangitis

    c. Bovine farcy

    d. Sporadic lymphangitis

23. **The causative agent for equine farcy is:**

    a. *Pseudomonas mallei*

    b. *Mycobacterium tuberculosis*

    c. *Nocardia farcinica*

    d. *Histomonas meleagridis*

24. **The causative agent for bovine farcy is:**

    a. *Pseudomonas mallei*

    b. *Mycobacterium tuberculosis*

    c. *Nocardia farcinica*

    d. *Histomonas meleagridis*

25. **The drug of choice for liver fluke infection in ruminants is:**

    a. Parental pamoate

    b. Oxyclozanide

    c. Piperazine

    d. Griseofulvin

26. **Which of the following drugs is used for the treatment of surra?**

    a. Quinapyramine sulphate + Quinapyramine chloride

    b. Quinapyramine sulphate + diaminazine aceturate

    c. Quinapyramine chloride + diaminazine aceturate

    d. Diaminazine aceturate + lithium antimony tartarate

27. **Dourine is caused by:**

    a. *Leishmania donovani*

    b. *Leishmania tropica*

    c. *Trypanosoma vivax*

    d. *Trypanosoma equiperdum*

28.   **In a blood smear, the *Trypanosoma* organism is found in the:**

    a. RBC

    b. Lymphocytes

    c. Platelets

    d. Plasma

29.   **A common complication of strangles in horses is:**

    a. Bastard strangles/metastatic infection

    b. Suppurative meningitis

    c. Suppurative necrotic bronchopneumonia

    d. All of these

30.   **During necropsy, the lamellated appearance of a pus-filled abscess inside the superficial lymph nodes in sheep is a characteristic finding of:**

    a. Tuberculosis

    b. Caseous lymphadenitis

    c. Ulcerative lymphangitis

    d. b and c

31.   **Ulcerative lymphangitis in cattle and horse is caused by:**

    a. *Corynebacterium pseudotuberculosis* biotype 1

    b. *Corynebacterium pseudotuberculosis* biotype 2

    c. a and b

    d. *Streptococcus bovis*

32.   **In a horse suffering from ulcerative lymphangitis, subcutaneous nodules and ulcers are usually restricted to which part of the body?**

    a. Neck

    b. Sub-mandibular region

c. Oral cavity

d. Lower limb

33. **Which of the following species are resistant to anthrax?**

a. Algerian sheep

b. Dwarf pigs

c. Dogs and cats

d. All of these

34. **A 'blackberry jam' consistency of the spleen is found in:**

a. Anthrax

b. Tuberculosis

c. Paratuberculosis

d. CBPP

35. **Which of the following samples can be collected to confirm the diagnosis of anthrax on an unopened carcass?**

a. Local oedema fluid

b. Peripheral blood

c. a and b

d. None of these

36. **Bubbly blood-stained salivation in cattle is a characteristic clinical sign of:**

a. FMD

b. Rinderpest

c. BVD-MD

d. Vesicular stomatitis

37. **The species most susceptible to PPR virus is:**

a. Goats

b. Cattle

c. Buffalo

d. Sheep

38. **At what age are goats the most susceptible to peste des petits ruminants (PPR)?**

    a. Younger than 2 months

    b. 2–4 months

    c. 4 months to 1 year

    d. 1–2 years

39. **The causative agent of malignant catarrhal fever (MCF) is:**

    a. Alphaherpesvirinae

    b. Betaherpesvirinae

    c. Gammaherpesvirinae

    d. All of these

40. **In the head and eye form of MCF, opacity of the cornea commences from the:**

    a. Centre of cornea

    b. Periphery of cornea

    c. Corneo–scleral junction

    d. Sclera

41. **The vector commonly responsible for biological transmission of bluetongue virus is:**

    a. Culicoides

    b. Mosquitoes

    c. Stomoxys

    d. Melophagus

42. **Which of the following is not a clinical manifestation of bluetongue in sheep?**

    a. Necrotic ulcers on the lateral aspect of the tongue

    b. Dark red to purple band on the skin just above the coronet

    c. Mucopurulent nasal discharge

    d. None of these

43.   **Pipe stem faeces in bovines is caused by:**

a. *Babesia bigemina*

b. *Babesia bovis*

c. *Babesia divergens*

d. All of these

44.   **Cerebral babesiosis in cattle is caused by:**

a. *B. bovis*

b. *B. bigemina*

c. *B. divergens*

d. *B. major*

45.   **East Coast fever is caused by:**

a. *Theileria sergenti*

b. *Theileria parva*

c. *Theileria annulata*

d. *Theileria hirci*

46.   **Punched out necrotic ulcers in the abomasum are the pathognomic lesions of which disease in calves?**

a. Theileriosis

b. Babesiosis

c. Anaplasmosis

d. Trypanosomosis

47.   **The dose of buparvaquone for the treatment of theileriosis is:**

a. 2.5 mg/kg

b. 5 mg/kg

c. 10 mg/kg

d. 20 mg/kg

48. **Dourine in horses is caused by:**

   a. *Trypanosoma evansi*

   b. *Trypanosoma congolense*

   c. *Trypanosoma cruzi*

   d. *Trypanosoma equiperdum*

49. **Which of the following is preferred for the detection of the *Trypanosoma* organism?**

   a. Thin blood smear

   b. Thick blood smear

   c. Plasma

   d. Lymph node aspirate

50. **'Silver dollar spot' on the body and neck is a characteristic finding of:**

   a. Cutaneous leishmaniasis

   b. Bovine lymphosarcoma

   c. Dourine

   d. Lumpy skin disease

51. **A 'rat tail' appearance in cattle can be seen in which of the following protozoal diseases?**

   a. Cutaneous leishmaniasis

   b. Coccidiosis

   c. Sarcocystosis

   d. Neosporosis

52. **Which of the following is not a differential of caprine arthritis encephalitis (CAE)?**

   a. Enzootic ataxia

   b. Spinal cord abscess

   c. Cerebrospinal nematodiasis

   d. Generalized neuropathy

53. **'Harder udder' syndrome, attributed to CAE virus infection, is characterized by:**

    a. Firm, swollen mammary glands and agalactia at the time of parturition

    b. Firm, swollen mammary glands with oozing straw-coloured fluid

    c. Firm, swollen udder and blood in milk at the time of parturition

    d. Swollen udder with normal milk production

54. **Clinical signs such as vesicles on the lips, muzzle, dental pad, tongue, gingivae, interdigital spaces and teats, and reluctance to eat and walk, are common in cows/buffalo with:**

    a. FMD

    b. IBR

    c. BVD

    d. MDC

55. **Which of the following is not a sign of PPR in goats?**

    a. Oculo-nasal discharge

    b. Diarrhoea and dehydration

    c. Sore mouth with swollen lips

    d. Swelling of knee joints

56. **Signs of equine infectious anaemia include:**

    a. Severe, persistent, bloody diarrhoea

    b. Intermittent fever and oedema of ventral abdomen and legs

    c. Frequent urination; urine containing large quantities of blood

    d. Bleeding from orifices

57. **Concerning management of a case of anthrax in a cow, which of the following steps is not recommended?**

    a. Don't report the disease to the authorities

    b. Vaccinate all food animals against anthrax

    c. Always do a complete necropsy

    d. Bury/or burn the carcass as soon as possible after diagnosis

58. Which of the following is an infectious but not a contagious disease?

a. Leptospirosis

b. Tetanus

c. Mucosal disease complex

d. Brucellosis

59. Endotoxaemia is a major cause of death in buffalo suffering from:

a. Black quarters

b. Haemorrhagic septicaemia

c. Black disease

d. Anaphylaxis

60. Primary vaccination of PPR in kids is performed at:

a. 3 months

b. 4 months

c. 5 months

d. 6 months

61. The Livaditis procedure is used for the diagnosis of:

a. Leptospirosis

b. Anaplasmosis

c. Ehrlichiosis

d. Lister

62. Which of the following diseases in cattle is caused by a retrovirus?

a. Bovine malignant catarrh

b. Bovine viral diarrhoea

c. Bovine leukosis

d. Rinderpest

63. **Potomac horse fever is caused by:**

   a. *Ehrlichia equi*

   b. *Ehrlichia risticii*

   c. *Ehrlichia ondiri*

   d. *Ehrlichia canis*

64. **Which of the following is the treatment of choice for chlamydiosis in goats?**

   a. Sulphonamide

   b. Fluoroquinolones

   c. Aminoglycosides

   d. Tetracycline

65. **Which of the following diseases is contagious in horses?**

   a. Tetanus

   b. Verminous colic

   c. Glanders

   d. Ascariasis

66. **Vegetative endocarditis is the chief lesion found in:**

   a. Classical swine fever

   b. African swine fever

   c. Swine erysipelas

   d. PRRS

67. **A mare should be vaccinated for viral rhinopneumonitis at which stages (month) of pregnancy?**

   a. 1st, 2nd and 3rd

   b. 4th, 5th and 6th

   c. 5th, 7th and 9th

   d. 4th, 6th and 8th

68. **Necrotizing myositis is the pathognomic lesion in which of the following diseases?**

    a. FMD

    b. BQ

    c. Anthrax

    d. Brucellosis

69. **Flaccid paralysis in botulism is caused by:**

    a. Inhibition of GABA

    b. Inhibition of glycine

    c. Inhibition of acetyl choline

    d. None of these

70. **Spastic paralysis in tetanus is caused by:**

    a. Inhibition of GABA

    b. Inhibition of glycine

    c. Inhibition of acetyl choline

    d. None of these

71. **Haemorrhagic septicaemia is more common in which species?**

    a. Cattle

    b. Buffalo

    c. Sheep

    d. Goats

72. **Benign tuberculosis is common in which species?**

    a. Cattle

    b. Pigs

    c. Goats

    d. Horses

73. **The Stormont test is used for the diagnosis of**

a. Tuberculosis

b. Paratuberculosis

c. Anthrax

d. Brucellosis

74. **An 'onion ring' appearance of the lymph nodes in sheep is a characteristic lesion of:**

a. Maedi-visna

b. Caseous lymphadenitis

c. Epizootic lymphangitis

d. None of these

75. **Which is a common clinical sign in cattle infected with pseudorabies?**

a. Convulsion

b. Bellowing

c. Pruritus

d. Abortion

76. **Infectious bovine rhinotracheitis is highly fatal in:**

a. Kids

b. Lambs

c. Calves

d. Adults

77. **Which of these species is a reservoir host for swine fever?**

a. Domestic pigs

b. Feral pigs

c. Ticks

d. Bats

78. **African swine fever is transmitted by:**

   a. Ticks

   b. Flies

   c. Earthworm

   d. Lice

79. **An amplifier host for Japanese encephalitis is:**

   a. Cattle

   b. Buffalo

   c. Sheep

   d. Pigs

80. **Which of the following is not a form of bovine malignant ca-tarrh?**

   a. Head and eye

   b. Alimentary

   c. Per-acute

   d. Cutaneous

81. **Animals vaccinated against anthrax should be withheld from slaughter for:**

   a. 90 days

   b. 60 days

   c. 45 days

   d. 7 days

82. **Listeriosis mostly occurs in which species?**

   a. Cattle

   b. Sheep

   c. Goats

   d. Horses

83. **Circling movements, head tilt, unilateral facial hypalgesia and facial paralysis in sheep are features of:**

   a. Ovine ketosis

   b. Enterotoxaemia

   c. Silage sickness

   d. Botulism

84. **Microabscessation of the CNS is the histological feature of which disease?**

   a. Rabies

   b. Listeriosis

   c. Botulism

   d. Bovine spongiform encephalopathy

85. **Sudden death, diamond-shaped skin lesions, arthritis and endocarditis in swine are characteristic features of:**

   a. Classical swine fever

   b. African swine fever

   c. Swine erysipelas

   d. Hog cholera

86. **Which of the following is not a symptom of lumpy jaw in cattle?**

   a. Rarefying osteomyelitis of mandible and maxilla

   b. Bony swellings, painful initially and painless in later stages

   c. Honey-like pus containing yellow-white granules

   d. Difficulty in mastication due to pain and mal-alignment of teeth in affected bone

87. **Sarcoid in horses is caused by which virus?**

   a. Cowpox

   b. Parapox

   c. Capripox

   d. Bovine papilloma

88. **Cauliflower-like warts in cattle is a characteristic feature of:**

    a. Lumpy skin disease

    b. Bovine papillomatosis

    c. Sarcoid

    d. All of these

89. **Which strain of rabies virus is considered a vaccine strain?**

    a. Street virus

    b. Fixed virus

    c. a and b

    d. None of these

90. **Which of the following species is considered a subclinical carrier of rabies?**

    a. Bats

    b. Foxes

    c. Mongooses

    d. Dogs

91. **Death in rabies commonly occurs due to:**

    a. Damage to the brain

    b. Respiratory paralysis

    c. Circulatory failure

    d. Syncope

92. **Which of the following tests is considered confirmatory for rabies?**

    a. RIA

    b. AGID

    c. FAT

    d. IFA

93. **Negri bodies are most commonly found in which part of the brain in rabies-infected cattle?**

    a. Hippocampus

    b. Purkinje cells of the cerebellum

    c. Grey matter of cerebrum

    d. Hypothalamus

94. **Bovine ephemeral fever is of what type?**

    a. Intermittent

    b. Remittent

    c. Biphasic

    d. Persistent

95. **Which of the following conditions is a feature of bovine ephemeral fever?**

    a. Secondary hypocalcaemia

    b. Serofibrinous polyserositis

    c. Accumulation of neutrophils in synovial fluid

    d. All of these

96. **Which of the following protozoal organisms is associated with endemic and epidemic abortion in cattle?**

    a. *Sarcocystis*

    b. *Neospora*

    c. *Trypanosoma*

    d. *Eimeria*

97. **Equine protozoal myeloencephalitis is caused by:**

    a. *Trypanosoma evansi*

    b. *Sarcocystis neurona*

    c. *Babesia equi*

    d. *Theileria equi*

98. **The dose of amprolium for the treatment of coccidiosis in calves is:**

   a. 5 mg/kg

   b. 10 mg/kg

   c. 15 mg/kg

   d. 20 mg/kg

99. **Which of the following organisms is responsible for development of lung cysts in cattle?**

   a. *Taenia saginatta*

   b. *Echinococcus granulosus*

   c. *Anoplocephala perfoliata*

   d. *Moniezia benedeni*

100. **Which organ is usually not affected in sheep with actinobacillosis?**

   a. Tongue

   b. Lower jaw

   c. Nose

   d. Face

101. **Pearl disease is also called:**

   a. Brucellosis

   b. Tuberculosis

   c. Paratuberculosis

   d. Dermatophytosis

102. **In an SID test for the detection of tuberculosis, the affected animal shows which type of hypersensitivity reaction?**

   a. Type I

   b. Type II

   c. Type III

   d. Type IV

103. **Which species is most commonly affected by Johne's disease?**

    a. Cattle

    b. Buffalo

    c. Sheep

    d. Goats

104. **Thick pea-soup-like faeces without any offensive odour is a symptom of:**

    a. Johne's disease

    b. Fasciolosis

    c. Salmonellosis

    d. Coccidiosis

105. **A thickened intestinal wall with corrugated mucosa is a characteristic necropsy finding for which disease?**

    a. Haemonchosis

    b. Paratuberculosis

    c. Coccidiosis

    d. Clostridial infection

106. **Strawberry foot rot in sheep is caused by:**

    a. *Staphylococcus aureus*

    b. *Dermatophillus congolensis*

    c. *Staphylococcus hyicus*

    d. *Streptococcus pyogenes*

107. **A horse is presented with purulent blood-stained nasal discharge with laboured breathing, discharge of dark honey-coloured pus from the skin nodules and thickened lymph vessels radiating from skin lesions. Which disease is most likely to be responsible?**

    a. Strangles

    b. Glanders

c. Ulcerative lymphangitis

d. Epizootic lymphangitis

108. **A mallein test is performed in the diagnosis of:**

a. Melioidosis

b. Caseous lymphadenitis

c. Glanders

d. Ulcerative lymphangitis

109. **Primary vaccination for classical swine fever is performed at what age?**

a. 3 months

b. 4 months

c. 5 months

d. 6 months

110. **Which parasite is a major cause of colic in equines?**

a. *Strongylus vulgaris*

b. *Oxyuris equi*

c. *Gasterophilus intestinalis*

d. *Parascaris equorum*

111. **Gall sickness is a synonym of :**

a. Babesiosis

b. Anaplasmosis

c. Trypanosomosis

d. None of these

112. **Pizzle rot in sheep is caused by:**

a. *Staphylococcus aureus*

b. *E. coli*

c. *Corynebacterium renale*

d. *Streptococcus uberis*

113. **Periodic ophthalmia in horses is seen in:**

    a. Leptospiral infection

    b. Listerial infection

    c. Glanders

    d. Equine protozoal myeloencephalitis

114. **A rectal pinch test is used in the diagnosis of:**

    a. Coccidiosis

    b. Paratuberculosis

    c. Salmonellosis

    d. Colibacillosis

115. **Lamsiekte in cattle and sheep is caused by:**

    a. *Clostridium botulinum* type A

    b. *Clostridium botulinum* type B

    c. *Clostridium botulinum* type C

    d. *Clostridium botulinum* type D

116. **Dunkop and dikkop are two forms of:**

    a. African swine fever

    b. Classical swine fever

    c. African horse sickness

    d. None of these

117. **Para-anthrax in pigs is caused by:**

    a. *Clostridium botulinum*

    b. *Clostridium septicum*

    c. *Clostridium hemolyticum*

    d. *Clostridium novyi*

118. **The site of intradermal injection in a mallein test is the:**

    a. Neck

    b. Lower eyelid

c. Base of tail

d. None of these

119. **The source of leptospirosis infection is:**

a. Infected urine

b. Uterine discharge

c. Aborted fetus

d. All of these

120. **Which type of nephritis is characteristic of leptospirosis?**

a. Glomerulonephritis

b. Interstitial nephritis

c. Pyelonephritis

d. All of these

121. **Which level of MAT titer of is considered positive for lepto-spiral infection?**

a. $\geq 1:10$

b. $\geq 1:20$

c. $\geq 1:50$

d. $\geq 1:100$

122. **Septicaemic pasteurellosis of cattle is associated with which infection?**

a. *Pasteurella multocida* biotype A

b. *Pasteurella multocida* biotype B

c. *Pasteurella hemolytica*

d. None of these

123. **Which serotype of *P. multocida* causes most outbreaks of haemorrhagic septicaemia in India?**

a. B1

b. B2

c. D

d. E2

124. **Which serotype of aphthovirus no longer causes FMD outbreaks?**

    a. A

    b. O

    c. C

    d. Asia-1

125. **The most common route of transmission for FMD virus in pigs is:**

    a. Ingestion

    b. Inhalation

    c. Cutaneous

    d. Vector

126. **Which of the following species is not susceptible to foot and mouth disease?**

    a. Elephants

    b. Deer

    c. Horses

    d. All of these

127. **'Hairy panters' is a common sequel to which disease in cattle?**

    a. Foot and mouth disease

    b. Malignant catarrhal fever

    c. Bovine respiratory disease complex

    d. Infectious bovine rhinotracheitis

128. **Button-shaped ulcers in the colonic mucosa of pigs are a characteristic necropsy finding in:**

    a. Classical swine fever

    b. African swine fever

    c. Transmissible gastroenteritis

    d. PRRS

129. **Viral replication in equine infectious anaemia occurs in:**

a. RBCs

b. Tissue macrophages

c. Myeloblast

d. Lymphocytes

130. **Which of the following is a pathological abnormality in equine infectious anaemia?**

a. Thrombocytopenia

b. Normocytic normochromic anaemia

c. Presence of sideroleukocytes

d. All of these

131. **Bovine spongiform encephalopathy in cattle is caused by:**

a. Virus

b. Cyanobacteria

c. Prion

d. Yeast

132. **Trismus with restricted jaw movement and a saw-horse posture are characteristic symptoms of:**

a. Actinobacillosis

b. Listeriosis

c. Tetanus

d. Enterotoxaemia

133. **Development of pustular and scabby lesions on the muzzle and lips of sheep and goats is characteristic of:**

a. PPR

b. Orf

c. Bluetongue

d. Rinderpest

134. **Which is the predilection site for *Brucella abortus*?**

    a. Testicles

    b. Pregnant uterus

    c. Udder

    d. All of these

135. **Bovine viral diarrhoea is antigenically related to which virus?**

    a. PPR

    b. Hog cholera

    c. Canine distemper

    d. All of these

136. **Which is the correct disinfectant formulation for foot and mouth disease?**

    a. 1–2% sodium hydroxide

    b. 4% sodium carbonate

    c. 1–2% formalin

    d. All these

137. **Sulphur granules in pus are seen in:**

    a. Strangles

    b. Actinobacillosis

    c. Actinomycosis

    d. b and c

138. **False black leg in sheep is associated with:**

    a. *Clostridium septicum*

    b. *Clostridium novyi*

    c. *Clostridium chauvoei*

    d. a and b

139. **A Coggins test is used in the diagnosis of:**

    a. African horse sickness

    b. Equine influenza

c. Equine infectious anaemia

d. Equine viral rhinopneumonitis

140. Haemorrhagic septicaemia is characterized by:

a. Sudden onset of fever

b. Severe dyspnea

c. Painful swelling of dewlap and brisket

d. All of these

141. In animals infected with brucellosis, which substance produced by the fetus is responsible for the growth of *Brucella abortus*?

a. Mycolic acid

b. Erythritol

c. Alpha-hydroxylase

d. Beta-hydroxylase

142. Abortion due to brucellosis principally occurs during which period of pregnancy?

a. First 3 months

b. Last 3 months

c. Mid-term

d. At any time

143. Strain 19 and strain RB51 vaccines are used to immunize against which disease?

a. Anthrax

b. Brucellosis

c. Trypanosomiasis

d. Black quarter

144. Calfhood vaccination is associated with which disease?

a. FMD

b. Anthrax

c. Brucellosis

d. Rabies

145. In cattle, the most common route of anthrax transmission is:

a. Ingestion

b. Inhalation

c. Cutaneous

d. All of these

146. Death in tetanus occurs due to:

a. Anoxia

b. Asphyxia

c. Septicaemia

d. Anuria

147. Hotis test is used to diagnose:

a. Mastitis

b. Equine infectious anaemia

c. Brucellosis

d. Salmonellosis

148. Pseudo FMD is also known as:

a. Vesicular exanthema

b. Bovine viral diarrhoea

c. Vesicular stomatitis

d. PPR

149. Which of the following organs is commonly affected in bovine leukosis?

a. Liver

b. Spinal cord

c. Brain

d. Lymph nodes

150.   In rabies, bellowing is commonly seen in which species:

   a. Sheep

   b. Cattle

   c. Horses

   d. Dogs

151.   The rabies virus is found in saliva and the:

   a. Olfactory nerve

   b. Salivary duct

   c. Optic nerve

   d. Respiratory mucosa

152.   Enterotoxaemia is a disease affecting:

   a. Sheep

   b. Lambs

   c. Cattle

   d. All ruminants

153.   Tuberculous lymphadenitis is characteristic of tuberculosis in which species?

   a. Pigs

   b. Sheep

   c. Horses

   d. None of these

154.   Turkey egg kidney in swine is a characteristic feature of:

   a. Picorna virus

   b. Pesti virus

   c. Lyssa virus

   d. Corona virus

155.   The amplifier host for FMD is:

   a. Cattle

   b. Deer

c. Pigs

d. Horses

156. Ringworm infection is transmitted through:

a. Direct contact

b. Ingestion

c. Aerosol

d. Inhalation

157. In dermatophytosis, which part of the skin is most commonly affected?

a. Stratum corneum

b. Stratum spinosum

c. Stratum basale

d. None of these

158. The Wood's lamp test is used in the diagnosis of:

a. Listeriosis

b. Dermatophytosis

c. Dermatophilosis

d. Histoplasmosis

159. Skin lesions caused by dermatophilosis in sheep have which appearance?

a. Palisade

b. Paintbrush

c. Vesicular

d. Nodular

160. Which of the following media is used to grow fungus?

a. Blood agar

b. Sabaoraud dextrose agar

c. Nutrient agar

d. BHI agar

161. **Aspergillosis in cattle is characterized by:**

    a. Abortion

    b. Pneumonia

    c. Mastitis

    d. All of these

162. **Aphthous fever is also known as:**

    a. FMD

    b. Vesicular stomatitis

    c. Vesicular exanthema

    d. Papillomatosis

163. **The juvenile form of bovine leukosis is seen in calves in which age group?**

    a. Less than 3 months

    b. 3 months to 6 months

    c. 6 months to 1 year

    d. Within 10 days of birth

164. **Abortion storm in cattle is caused by:**

    a. *Leptospira Pomona*

    b. *Leptospira hardzo*

    c. *Leptospira icterohemorrhagica*

    d. *Leptospira grippotyphosa*

165. **Cold mastitis is caused by:**

    a. *Staphylococcus* spp.

    b. *Streptococcus* spp.

    c. *Leptospira* spp.

    d. *Mycoplasma* spp.

166. **In tetanus-affected animals, death occurs due to:**

    a. Anoxia

    b. Coma

c. Syncope

d. Asphyxia

167. **In a healthy lactating mammary gland, the somatic cell count (SCC) is:**

   a. < 100 cells/ml

   b. < 1000 cells/ml

   c. < 1,00,000 cells/ml

   d. < 10,00,000 cells/ml

168. **An organism not commonly associated with contagious mastitis is:**

   a. *Streptococcus agalactiae*

   b. *Streptococcus dysgalactiae*

   c. *Mycobacterium bovis*

   d. *Staphylococcus aureus*

169. **The most reliable cowside test for detecting subclinical mastitis is:**

   a. Hotis

   b. CMT

   c. NAGase

   d. White side

170. **A wheelbarrow test is recommended for the diagnosis of:**

   a. Scrapie

   b. Ovine pulmonary adenomatosis

   c. Louping ill

   d. Maedi-visna

171. **Transmissible gastroenteritis in pigs is caused by which virus?**

   a. Rota virus

   b. Corona virus

c. Adeno virus

d. Varicella virus

172. PPR virus has an affinity towards which tissue?

a. Epithelial

b. Lymphoid

c. Epidermis

d. None of these

173. Biliary fever in horses is caused by:

a. *Ehrlichia*

b. *Babesia*

c. *Theileria*

d. *Cowdria*

174. Pseudorabies is caused by which virus?

a. Rhabdo virus

b. Herpes virus

c. Adeno virus

d. Flavi virus

175. Intracytoplasmic vacuolation of brain neurons occurs in which disease?

a. Scrapie

b. Bovine spongiform encephalitis

c. a and b

d. None of these

176. The prophylactic dose of tetanus antitoxin serum in cattle and horses is:

a. 1500–3000 IU I/M

b. 5000 IU I/M

c. 1 lac IU I/M

d. 10 lac IU I/M

177. **Which disease is characterized by abortion, fever, anaemia, hemoglobinuria and icterus?**

    a. Hemorrhagic septicaemia

    b. Glanders

    c. Listeriosis

    d. Leptospirosis

178. **Which disease in sheep causes the lungs to become rubbery?**

    a. Maedi

    b. Jaagsiekte

    c. a and b

    d. None of these

179. **Which species is resistant to tuberculosis?**

    a. Cattle

    b. Goats

    c. Horses

    d. Buffalo

180. **In which disease are picnotic changes in the nucleus of epithelial cells found?**

    a. FMD

    b. RP

    c. a and b

    d. Ephemeral fever

181. **Heartwater disease is caused by:**

    a. *Cowdria ruminantium*

    b. *Moraxella bovis*

    c. Equine influenza virus

    d. All of these

182. **Which disease leads to abortion in late pregnancy?**

    a. Trichomoniasis

    b. Vibriosis

    c. Mycotic diseases

    d. Listeriosis

183. **The biliary form of babesiosis is common in which species?**

    a. Cattle

    b. Poultry

    c. Horses

    d. Dogs

184. **In which of the following species is haemoglobinuria not a feature in babesiosis?**

    a. Sheep

    b. Cattle

    c. Horses

    d. Dogs

185. **The effective incubation temperature for fungal growth in SDA is:**

    a. 25 °C

    b. 37 °C

    c. 50 °C

    d. 21 °C

186. **Thrush is a fungal disease observed in:**

    a. Cattle

    b. Sheep

    c. Poultry

    d. All of these

187. **Sporotrichosis mainly occurs in:**

   a. Cattle

   b. Dogs

   c. Horses

   d. Pigs

188. **A rat-tailed appearance in horses occurs due to infection with:**

   a. *Strongylus vulgaris*

   b. *Oxyuris equi*

   c. *Parascaris equorum*

   d. *Ascaris suum*

189. **'Biting its own body' is a peculiar feature of rabies in which species?**

   a. Swine

   b. Cattle

   c. Dogs

   d. Horses

190. **Which disease is characterized by intermittent fever?**

   a. Anthrax

   b. Rabies

   c. Equine influenza

   d. Equine infectious anaemia

191. **In which disease are the mesodermal tissues (joints, muscles, lymph nodes) affected?**

   a. Ephemeral fever

   b. Bluetongue

   c. African horse sickness

   d. All of these

192. **Which of the following are stages of pox lesion?**

a. Erythema–Papule–Pustule–Blister

b. Erythema–Pustule–Vesicle–Papule–Blister

c. Erythema–Papule–Vesicle–Pustule–Blister

d. None of these

193. **Renal failure is a cause of death in which disease?**

a. Leptospirosis

b. Listeriosis

c. Salmonellosis

d. Glanders

194. **Encephalitis, abortion, endometritis and repeat breeding are characteristic symptoms of:**

a. Listeriosis

b. Glanders

c. Leptospirosis

d. Salmonellosis

195. **The case fatality rate in BQ is:**

a. 100%

b. 70%

c. 30%

d. 0%

196. **Toxins of *Clostridium tetani* include:**

a. Exotoxin

b. Neurotoxin

c. Endotoxin

d. All of these

197. **Early rigor mortis is an important post-mortem finding in:**

a. Enterotoxemia

b. Anthrax

    c. Tetanus

    d. Strangles

198. **Unilateral facial paralysis occurs in:**

    a. Listeriosis

    b. Glanders

    c. Leptospirosis

    d. Salmonellosis

199. **Which of the following is a veneral disease of cattle?**

    a. Actinobacillosis

    b. Actinomycosis

    c. Campylobacteriosis

    d. All of these

200. **In cattle, osteomyelitis and rarefication of the mandible occurs in:**

    a. Actinobacillosis

    b. Actinomycosis

    c. Campylobacteriosis

    d. All of these

.

Answers

1.	a	31.	b	61.	a	91.	b
2.	b	32.	d	62.	c	92.	c
3.	d	33.	d	63.	b	93.	b
4.	b	34.	a	64.	d	94.	c
5.	c	35.	c	65.	c	95.	d
6.	b	36.	b	66.	c	96.	b
7.	c	37.	a	67.	c	97.	b
8.	b	38.	c	68.	b	98.	b
9.	b	39.	c	69.	c	99.	b
10.	c	40.	c	70.	a	100.	a
11.	c	41.	a	71.	b	101.	b
12.	d	42.	d	72.	b	102.	d
13.	a	43.	c	73.	a	103.	a
14.	a	44.	b	74.	b	104.	a
15.	d	45.	b	75.	c	105.	b
16.	c	46.	a	76.	c	106.	b
17.	b	47.	a	77.	b	107.	b
18.	a	48.	d	78.	a	108.	c
19.	b	49.	b	79.	d	109.	a
20.	b	50.	c	80.	d	110.	a
21.	b	51.	c	81.	c	111.	b
22.	a	52.	d	82.	b	112.	c
23.	a	53.	a	83.	c	113.	a
24.	c	54.	a	84.	b	114.	b
25.	b	55.	d	85.	c	115.	d
26.	a	56.	b	86.	b	116.	c
27.	d	57.	c	87.	d	117.	b
28.	d	58.	b	88.	b	118.	b
29.	d	59.	b	89.	b	119.	d
30.	b	60.	a	90.	a	120.	b

(Continued)

121.	d	141.	b	161.	d	181.	a
122.	b	142.	b	162.	a	182.	a
123.	b	143.	b	163.	b	183.	c
124.	c	144.	c	164.	a	184.	c
125.	a	145.	a	165.	c	185.	b
126.	c	146.	b	166.	d	186.	d
127.	a	147.	a	167.	c	187.	c
128.	a	148.	c	168.	b	188.	b
129.	b	149.	d	169.	b	189.	d
130.	d	150.	b	170.	b	190.	d
131.	c	151.	a	171.	b	191.	a
132.	c	152.	c	172.	b	192.	c
133.	b	153.	a	173.	b	193.	a
134.	d	154.	b	174.	a	194.	a
135.	b	155.	c	175.	a	195.	a
136.	d	156.	a	176.	a	196.	b
137.	d	157.	a	177.	d	197.	c
138.	d	158.	b	178.	a	198.	a
139.	b	159.	b	179.	b	199.	c
140.	d	160.	b	180.	a	200.	b

2 Viral Diseases

J.B. Kathiriya and Chetan Chavda

Introduction

Infectious diseases of farm animals are a major threat to agriculture and can cause great damage in both industrialized and developing countries. In the last two centuries considerable effort has been invested in understanding the causes and pathogenesis of viral and bacterial diseases in domestic animals.

The questions in this chapter cover the important viral diseases of farm animals, including cattle, buffalo, sheep, goats, pigs and poultry.

© CAB International 2024. *Key Questions in Preventative Farm Animal Medicine Volume 1: Types, Causes and Treatment of Infectious Diseases* (ed. T. Rana)
DOI: 10.1079/9781800624726.0002

Multiple Choice Questions

1. **Which virus type is EDS?**

    a. Aviadenovirus

    b. Siadenovirus

    c. Adenovirus

    d. Atadenovirus

2. **Ephemeral fever is also known as:**

    a. 3-day fever

    b. Stiff sickness

    c. a and b

    d. None of these

3. **Severe vomiting, grey, foul-smelling diarrhoea and gastro-enteritis in pups are characteristics of:**

    a. Parvovirus

    b. Infectious canine hepatitis

    c. Canine distemper

    d. Rabies

4. **The rabies virus belongs to the genus:**

    a. Vesiculovirus

    b. Adenovirus

    c. Lyssavirus

    d. Novirhabdovirus

5. **Newcastle disease can be isolated in embryonated chicken eggs by which route of inoculation?**

    a. CAM

    b. Yolk sac

    c. Amniotic

    d. Allantoic

6.   **Pump handle respiration is a typical clinical sign observed in:**

   a. Infectious laryngotracheitis

   b. Infectious bronchitis

   c. Avian influenza

   d. Newcastle disease

7.   **Herpesvirus in turkeys is used as a vaccine for:**

   a. Marek's disease

   b. IBR

   c. ILT

   d. None of these

8.   **Swine fever virus can be propagated in:**

   a. MDBK

   b. Primary pig kidney cells

   c. Vero

   d. Primary calf kidney cells

9.   **Big liver disease is caused in:**

   a. ILT

   b. MD

   c. Avian leucosis complex

   d. ND

10.   **Equine encephalitis virus belongs to the family:**

   a. Birnaviridae

   b. Flaviviridae

   c. Togaviridae

   d. Calciviridae

11.   **Which virus family has a segmented genome?**

   a. Reoviridae

   b. Bunyaviridae

c. Birnaviridae

d. All of these

12. **Which of these viruses is neurotrophic?**

a. Rabies

b. Aujeszky's disease

c. a and b

d. None of these

13. **Pol genes in retroviruses encode for:**

a. Reverse transcriptase

b. Integrase

c. a and b

d. None of these

14. **Which cytopathic effects are seen in PPR infection?**

a. Acidophilic intracytoplasmic inclusion body formation

b. Syncytial formation

c. Inclusion bodies in cytoplasm and nucleus

d. All of these

15. **Persistent infection is seen in:**

a. Equine infectious anaemia

b. Rinderpest

c. Maedi-visna

d. a and b

16. **In which virus does the ribonucleoprotein have a herring-bone appearance?**

a. African horse sickness

b. Equine infectious anaemia

c. Equine influenza

d. None of these

17. **The lentogenic strain of Newcastle disease virus is called:**

    a. Komorow

    b. Hertz

    c. Milano

    d. La Sota

18. **Which is an example of cubical symmetry virus?**

    a. Orthomyxoviridae

    b. Rhabdoviridae

    c. Paramyxoviridae

    d. Picornaviridae

19. **Hard pad disease is caused by:**

    a. Morbillivirus

    b. Parvovirus

    c. Adenovirus

    d. Rotavirus

20. **Which of the following is the smallest virus?**

    a. Coronaviridae

    b. Togaviridae

    c. Retroviridae

    d. Circoviridae

21. **Which of the following is not antigenically related to the other three viruses?**

    a. Rinderpest

    b. Mumps

    c. CD virus

    d. Measles

22. **In which infection does corneal opacity in dogs develop?**

    a. Canine distemper

    b. Canine parvovirus

c. Rabies

d. Infectious canine hepatitis

23.   Which is the vaccine strain for infectious bronchitis?

a. Mukteswar

b. Massachusetts

c. La Sota

d. R2B

24.   Which is the biological vector in the transmission of African swine fever?

a. Culicids sp.

b. Ornithodorus sp.

c. a and b

d. None of these

25.   Milker's nodule is caused by:

a. Capripox

b. Parapox

c. Cowpox

d. Suipox

26.   The predilection site for parvovirus is:

a. Bone marrow

b. Enteric epithelium

c. Foetus

d. All these

27.   Cup-shaped depressions are seen in the surface of:

a. Calcivirus

b. Picornavirus

c. Togavirus

d. Parvovirus

28. **Antigenic shift is more common in:**

    a. Orthomyxoviruses

    b. Bunyaviruses

    c. Arenaviruses

    d. All of these

29. **These poxviruses are antigenically related except:**

    a. Cow pox

    b. Sheep pox

    c. Lumpy skin disease virus

    d. Goat pox

30. **Acyclovir is a drug of choice for:**

    a. Calicivirus infection

    b. Rhabdovirus infection

    c. Poxvirus infection

    d. Herpesvirus infection

31. **Interactions of viruses occurs by:**

    a. Carbohydrates

    b. Lipids

    c. Proteins

    d. Nucleic acid

32. **Infectious bovine rhinotracheitis virus belongs to which family?**

    a. Herpesviridae

    b. Togaviridae

    c. Poxiviridae

    d. None of these

33. **The nucleic acid of rinderpest virus is:**

    a. dsDNA

    b. dsRNA

c. ssDNA

d. ssRNA

34. **The nucleic acid of avian enterovirus causing avian encephalomyelitis is:**

a. ssDNA

b. dsRNA

c. dsDNA

d. ssRNA

35. **ICH virus belongs to which family?**

a. Hepatomaviridae

b. Adenoviridae

c. Herpesviridae

d. Picornaviridae

36. **Plague assay was introduced into animal virology by:**

a. Dulbecco

b. Bong

c. Rous

d. None of these

37. **Equine infectious anaemia virus belongs to which family?**

a. Retroviridae

b. Flaviviridae

c. Vegaviridae

d. None of these

38. **Idiotype is present in:**

a. Viral envelope

b. Viral nucleic acid

c. Variable region of antibodies

d. Constant region of antibodies

39. **Ether can inactivate:**

   a. Enveloped virus

   b. Non-enveloped virus

   c. a and b

   d. None of these

40. **Borna virus in equines belongs to which family?**

   a. Goroviridae

   b. Flaviviridae

   c. Picornaviridae

   d. Bornaviridae

41. **The causative agent of scrapie in sheep is:**

   a. Virioid

   b. Prion

   c. Virusoid

   d. All of these

42. **The genome for African swine fever is:**

   a. dsDNA

   b. dsRNA

   c. ssDNA

   d. ssRNA

43. **Which characteristic is held by members of the Birnaviridae family?**

   a. Enveloped

   b. Non-enveloped

   c. a and b

   d. None of these

44. **Antigenic variation in viruses was first identified in:**

    a. Tobacco mosaic virus

    b. FMD virus

    c. Rabies virus

    d. Rou's sarcoma virus

45. **Independent heredity transcription and translation in viruses is associated with:**

    a. dsDNA

    b. dsRNA

    c. ssDNA

    d. ssRNA

46. **Ring-shaped long capsomeres arranged in a hexagonal pattern showing 32 visible holes appear in:**

    a. Bunyavirus

    b. Calcivirus

    c. Rotavirus

    d. Coronavirus

47. **Viral nucleic acid extracted from heat-inactivated virus pre-parations is:**

    a. Antigenic

    b. Non-infectious

    c. Infectious

    d. None of these

48. **Viral protein capsid is a transcriptional product of:**

    a. Immediate early gene

    b. Delayed gene

    c. Delayed early gene

    d. Post-transcriptional process of mRNA

49. **What is the name for ssDNA virus?**

    a. Hepatitis B

    b. Parvovirus

    c. Bunyavirus

    d. None of these

50. **dsRNA segment genome is a characteristic feature of:**

    a. Paramyxovirus

    b. Retrovirus

    c. Orthomyxovirus

    d. Reovirus

51. **Which virus is the odd one out on the basis of its structure?**

    a. Adenovirus

    b. Popovavirus

    c. Picornavirus

    d. Coronavirus

52. **Viruses having a heterogenic effect belonged to which family?**

    a. Reoviridae

    b. Adenoviridae

    c. Herpesviridae

    d. Caluviridae

53. **Defective interfering virus particles interfere in the replication of:**

    a. Heterologous viruses

    b. Related viruses

    c. Homologous viruses

    d. None of these

54. **Which is a plasmid vector of *E. coli*?**

   a. PSE 101

   b. RWW 0

   c. RSF 1010

   d. None of these

55. **Equine herpesvirus-1 causes:**

   a. Respiratory neurological disease and abortion in mares

   b. Hepatic disease in equines

   c. a and b

   d. None of these

56. **The RNA of vascular exanthema virus in swine is:**

   a. Infectious

   b. Non-infectious

   c. a and b

   d. None of these

57. **Rinderpest can occur in camels and in its epidemiology:**

   a. Camels are important

   b. The role of camels is not known

   c. Camels do not play an important role

   d. None of these

58. **Wild animals are not important in the spread of:**

   a. Rinderpest

   b. PPR

   c. a and b

   d. None of these

59. **Which species is most susceptible to African horse sickness?**

   a. Horses

   b. Donkeys

c. Mules

d. Deer

60. **Bovine viral diarrhoea virus can be detected in cell cultures by:**

a. FAT

b. Viral interference

c. FAT & Viral interference

d. CPE

61. **Newcastle disease can cause which of the following in humans and cows:**

a. Conjunctivitis

b. Fatality

c. Diarrhoea

d. All of these

62. **Which cell culture is most sensitive for the isolation of FMD virus?**

a. Primary calf kidney

b. BHK-21

c. PK-15

d. Calf thyroid

63. **Most enveloped viruses are released by:**

a. Cell lysis

b. Endocytosis

c. Budding

d. None

64. **Viruses:**

a. Lack the enzymes necessary for protein and HA synthesis

b. Multiply by complex mechanisms

c. Multiply by binary fission

d. Are unaffected by antibacterial antibiotics

65. **The electron microscope was invented by:**

a. Antony van Leuwenhoek

b. Ruska

c. Elford

d. L. Pasteur

66. **Who first observed that FMD was caused by a filterable agent?**

a. Beijerinck

b. Walter Reed

c. Loeffler and Frosch

d. Edward Jenner

67. **The term vaccine was coined by:**

a. Robert Koch

b. J. Bordet

c. Zinke

d. L. Pasteur

68. **Who first produced tobacco mosaic disease by filterable agent?**

a. Stanley

b. Henle

c. Iwanowski

d. Twort

69. **Who first crystallized tobacco mosaic virus (TMV)?**

a. Berkfield

b. Stanley

c. Lindenmann

d. Kitosato

70. **The symmetric protein shell of viruses which encloses viral nucleic acid is known as the:**

    a. Envelope

    b. Capsomere

    c. Capsid

    d. Non-virulent

71. **Outside a host cell, uncoated virus nucleic acid is:**

    a. Infective

    b. Virulent

    c. Inert

    d. Non-virulent

72. **Which is incorrect concerning viruses?**

    a. They are unicellular organisms

    b. They contain DNA and RNA

    c. They are haploid in nature

    d. They multiply by binary fission ND

73. **Viruses:**

    a. Are susceptible to antibiotics

    b. Are susceptible to interferons

    c. May be grown in artificial media

    d. Can be seen under a light microscope

74. **The clear area resulting from virus multiplication on an agar overlay cell culture is known as a:**

    a. Pock

    b. Focal CPE

    c. Plague

    d. None of these

75.   **Ultrasonic waves release a virus from an infected cell by:**

a. Sailing the cell membrane

b. Disrupting the cell

c. Shrinking the cell

d. None of these

76.   **Which of the following viruses does not induce tumour formation?**

a. Retrovirus

b. Iridoviridae

c. Herpesvirus

d. Parvovirus

77.   **Which virus family does not induce malignant tumours in domestic animals?**

a. Retroviridae

b. Papovarvidae

c. Parvoviridae

d. Herpesviridae

78.   **How does papilloma virus produce carcinoma?**

a. Naturally

b. Experimentally

c. a and b

d. None of these

79.   **How does papilloma virus produce tumours?**

a. Naturally

b. Naturally and experimentally in infants

c. Experimentally in rodents

d. None of these

80.   **Adenoviruses produce tumours:**

a. Naturally

b. Experimentally in rodents

c. Naturally and experimentally in infants

d. All of these

81.   **Which viral infection does not occur via the skin?**

a. Pox disease

b. Tumour due to papilloma viruses

c. Herpesviruses

d. Bluetongue

82.   **The incubation period for infectious canine hepatitis is:**

a. 4–9 days

b. 2–3 weeks

c. 4 weeks

d. 5–6 weeks

83.   **ICH virus is excreted from the body via:**

a. Nasal discharge

b. Faeces

c. Urine

d. All of these

84.   **Which of the following laboratory animals is most suitable for the typing of FMD virus?**

a. Guinea pigs

b. Rats

c. Hamsters

d. Unweaned mice

85.   **Aphthovirus is typed using:**

a. ELISA

b. CDT

  c. Virus neutralization test

  d. All of these

86. **The most effective chemical disinfectant to kill FMD virus is:**

  a. 2% formalin

  b. 2% Sodium hypochlorite

  c. 70% alcohol

  d. 2% $Na_2 CO_3$

87. **An animal becomes infected by more than one type of aphthovirus due to:**

  a. Poor immunity

  b. Antigenic drift

  c. Antigen diversity

  d. All of these

88. **Haemagglutinins are :**

  a. Polysaccharides

  b. Glycoproteins

  c. Proteins

  d. Lipoproteins

89. **A haemagglutination test is given using:**

  a. Live viruses

  b. Dead viruses

  c. a and b

  d. None of these

90. **Freund's complete adjuvant contains a potent non-specific immunostimulant obtained from:**

  a. *M. leprae*

  b. *M. phlei*

  c. *C. parium*

  d. *E. coli*

91. **The incubation period for rabies in dogs in most cases is:**

a. 1–2 weeks

b. 3–6 months

c. 2–10 weeks

d. 6–12 months

92. **A rabid dog in 'dumb' form:**

a. Always bites

b. Seldom bites

c. Often bites

d. Never bites

93. **Which laboratory animal is most preferred for the isolation of street rabies?**

a. Rabbits

b. Suckling mice

c. Guinea pigs

d. White rats

94. **The sylvatic type of rabies Is transmitted by:**

a. Dogs

b. Wild animals

c. Domestic animals

d. Vampire bats

95. **In which media is rabies virus not secreted?**

a. Milk

b. Blood

c. Saliva

d. Tears

96. **In a rabies-endemic area, if a street dog has bitten a person the dog must be quarantined for:**

    a. At least 3 days

    b. At least 5 days

    c. At least 10 days

    d. At least 14 days

97. **What was the original source of the rabies Flurry strain?**

    a. Chickens

    b. Humans

    c. Dogs

    d. Rabbits

98. **Select a rabies vaccine that is free from post-vaccinal reactions:**

    a. Samples vaccine

    b. Mouse brain vaccine

    c. Duck embryo vaccine

    d. Human diploid cell culture vaccine

99. **What is the incubation period for Newcastle disease?**

    a. 1–2 days

    b. 2–3 days

    c. 5–6 days

    d. 2–3 months

100. **What is the incubation period for equine influenza virus?**

    a. 2 months

    b. 1–3 days

    c. 4 months

    d. 1–3 weeks

101. **What is the incubation period for PPR?**

a. 2–3 days

b. 2 months

c. 4–9 days

d. 1 month

102. **What is the incubation period for canine distemper?**

a. 5–8 days

b. 10 days

c. 2–4 days

d. 14 days

103. **What is the incubation period for foot and mouth disease?**

a. 1–2 weeks

b. 14 weeks

c. 2–4 days

d. 14 days

104. **What is the incubation period for rabies in humans?**

a. 21 days to 2–3 months

b. 14 days

c. 10 days

d. 1 year

105. **What is the incubation period for bluetongue disease?**

a. 6–7 days

b. 1 month

c. 2–3 days

d. 2 months

106. **What is the incubation period for rabies in dogs?**

a. 1–2 weeks

b. 14 weeks

   c. 3–10 weeks

   d. 28 weeks

107. **Both intranuclear and intracytoplasmic inclusion bodies are present in infections caused by:**

   a. Morbilli virus (Paramyxoviridae)

   b. Rabies virus

   c. CD virus

   d. IBH

108. **Double-stranded RNA is found in:**

   a. Retrovirus

   b. Poxvirus

   c. Reovirus

   d. Parvovirus

109. **The model virus for tumour research is:**

   a. Polyomavirus

   b. Rou's sarcoma virus

   c. Shope papilloma virus

   d. Reovirus

110. **In rabies, Negri bodies are seen in the:**

   a. Hippocampus and cerebrum

   b. Hippocampus and cerebellum

   c. Medulla and hippocampus

   d. Cerebrum and medulla

111. **Pseudorabies is caused by:**

   a. Lyssavirus

   b. Paramyxovirus

   c. Picornavirus

   d. Herpesvirus

112. **The mode of transmission for IBR virus is:**

    a. Venereal

    b. Inhalation

    c. a and b

    d. None of these

113. **Equine sarcoid is caused by:**

    a. Paramyxovirus

    b. Poxvirus

    c. Reovirus

    d. Papillomavirus

114. **Which of the following is not of the genus morbillivirus?**

    a. Measles

    b. CD

    c. ICH

    d. Rinderpest

115. **Which virus causes diffuse destruction of neurons through-out grey matter?**

    a. Equine viral arteritis

    b. Japanese B encephalitis

    c. Louping ill

    d. Bovine viral diarrhoea

116. **Which family causes infectious laryngotracheitis?**

    a. Herpesviridae

    b. Picornaviridae

    c. Poxiviridae

    d. Rotavirus

117. **ILT virus is mainly spread:**

    a. Horizontally

    b. Laterally

c. Vertically

d. All of these

118. **The causal organism for epidemic tremor is:**

a. Picornavirus

b. Adenovirus

c. Poxvirus

d. Paramyxovirus

119. **Outbreaks of ILT are mainly seen in which age group of birds?**

a. 5–9 months

b. 21 days

c. 3–4 months

d. All age groups

120. **What is the predisposing factor for severe ILT disease?**

a. Deficit of vitamin A

b. Excess ammonia in the atmosphere

c. a and b

d. Deficit of B complex

121. **The incubation period of ILT is:**

a. 6–12 days

b. 3–4 days

c. 20–24 days

d. None of these

122. **A characteristic feature of acute ILT is:**

a. Torticollis

b. Dyspnoea

c. Convulsion

d. Paralysis

123. **A sign of ILT is:**

   a. Moist rales

   b. Wide open mouth and gasping

   c. Bloodstained sputum

   d. All of these

124. **In cases of ILT, lesions are mainly seen in the:**

   a. Upper respiratory tract

   b. Lower respiratory tract

   c. Digestive system

   d. Genital system

125. **Which post-mortem sign indicates per acute ILT?**

   a. Haemorrhagic tracheitis

   b. Bloodstained mucous in trachea

   c. a and b

   d. Caseous diphtheritic exudate

126. **What is infectious avian encephalomyelitis also known as?**

   a. Aftosa

   b. Epidemic tremor

   c. Pink eye

   d. Wattles disease

127. **Which system is primarily affected in cases of epidemic tremor in young chicks?**

   a. Peripheral nervous

   b. Central nervous

   c. Musculoskeletal

   d. Respiratory

128. **Epidemic tremor is indicated by:**

   a. Ataxia

   b. Paralysis

c. Stunted growth

d. All of these

129. What is the incubation period of swine fever?

a. 1–2 weeks

b. 14 weeks

c. 3–10 weeks

d. 28 weeks

130. Which of these is a method of virus cultivation?

a. Cell culture

b. Agglutination test

c. Serological test

d. Milk ring test

131. The cell line for poxvirus is:

a. Hela cell line

b. MD BK

c. Liver cell

d. All of these

132. Transformed cells that do not die and are capable of multiplication for an indefinite period are known as:

a. Cell lines

b. Cell cultures

c. Secondary cell lines

d. All of these

133. Viruses can be stored for prolonged periods by:

a. Lyophilisation

b. Being frozen at −70 °C

c. Freeze drying

d. None of these

134. **Which virus is associated with the development of syncytia in a cell culture?**

    a. Aphthovirus

    b. Rinderpest

    c. Hog cholera virus

    d. Buffalo poxvirus

135. **Bluetongue virus is transmitted through:**

    a. Semen only

    b. Congenital mode only

    c. Arthropod bite only

    d. All of the above

136. **Which virus is capable of infecting and destroying the primary lymphoid organ?**

    a. Canine distemper

    b. Infectious bursal disease

    c. African swine fever

    d. BVD

137. **Adenoviruses are identified by the presence of:**

    a. Sand particles

    b. Lipid droplets

    c. Ribosomes

    d. All of these

138. **Embryonated eggs are used for virus cultivation over tissue culture because they are:**

    a. Easily available and cheap

    b. Manipulated with less effort

    c. Devoid of a natural defence system

    d. All of these

139. **An allantoic membrane is used for the cultivation of:**

    a. Toga virus

    b. Pox virus

    c. Myxo virus

    d. Influenza and mumps virus

140. **Which poultry disease is not caused by a virus:**

    a. Chronic respiratory disease

    b. Fowl pox

    c. Infectious bronchitis

    d. Ranikhet disease

141. **Which nucleic acid is present in viruses?**

    a. DNA

    b. RNA

    c. Either DNA or RNA

    d. Both DNA and RNA

142. **EDS-76 is:**

    a. Herpesvirus

    b. Coronavirus

    c. Adenovirus

    d. Poxvirus

143. **Bovine ephemeral fever virus belongs to the family:**

    a. Herpesviridae

    b. Rhabdoviridae

    c. Reoviridae

    d. Togaviridae

144. **Samples suspected for pox virus are inoculated in embryonated eggs by the route of:**

    a. Allantoic cavity

    b. Amniotic cavity

c. CAM

d. Yolk sac

145. **Which animals are not susceptible to vesicular exanthema virus?**

a. Pigs

b. Horses

c. Cows

d. All of these

146. **Which virus has a criss-cross pattern on its surface?**

a. Contagious pustular dermatitis virus

b. Fowl pox virus

c. Adenovirus

d. Parvovirus

147. **Which virus has cyclic DNA?**

a. Papovavirus

b. Parvovirus

c. Pestivirus

d. Poxvirus

148. **The diploid genome is characteristic of which virus family?**

a. Retroviridae

b. Rhabdoviridae

c. Reoviridae

d. None of these

149. **Bovine viral diarrhoea virus belongs to which family?**

a. Togaviridae

b. Reoviridae

c. Herpesviridae

d. Flaviviridae

150. **Which of the following is correctly matched?**

    a. Picornavirus–Ranikhet disease

    b. Lumpy skin disease–poxvirus

    c. Diamond skin disease–Herpesvirus

    d. Paramyxovirus–FMD

151. **Yellow fever is caused by:**

    a. Flavivirus

    b. Lyssavirus

    c. Hendravirus

    d. Picornavirus

152. **Yellow fever is transmitted by:**

    a. Aedes aegypti

    b. Argus

    c. Ioxides

    d. Simules

153. **The separation of RBCs from a virus is called:**

    a. Elution

    b. HA

    c. HI

    d. Eclipse

154. **Which viral agent produces diphasic fever, respiratory distress, nervous symptoms and hard pad disease in dogs?**

    a. Canine distemper

    b. ICH

    c. Rabies

    d. IBH

155. **Which virus has RNA-dependent DNA polymerase?**

    a. Retrovirus

    b. Reovirus

  c. Rabies virus

  d. Rubella virus

156. Chickenpox in man is caused by:

  a. Poxvirus

  b. Herpesvirus

  c. Adenovirus

  d. Parvovirus

157. The swine influenza virus associated with humans is:

  a. H1N1

  b. H2N2

  c. H3N2

  d. H5N1

158. Intranuclear inclusion bodies are seen in:

  a. Pox diseases

  b. Herpesvirus infection

  c. Adenovirus infection

  d. Lyssavirus infection

159. Negri bodies seen in rabies are:

  a. Intranuclear

  b. Intracytoplasmic

  c. a and b

  d. Intranuclear or intracytoplasmic

160. The source of 'reverse transcriptase' enzyme used for cDNA synthesis is:

  a. Moloney murine leukaemia virus

  b. (AMV)

  c. Both

  d. None of these

161. **Quantitative studies using PCR technique can be performed with:**

    a. RT-PCR

    b. Real-time PCR

    c. Micro array

    d. None of these

162. **Viruses that exist in cells and cause recurrent disease are considered:**

    a. Oncogenic

    b. Cytopathic

    c. Latent

    d. Resistant

163. **Which if these is not a morbillivirus?**

    a. Mumps

    b. Measles

    c. PPR

    d. Rinderpest

164. **Flaviviridae is:**

    a. dsDNA

    b. ds RNA

    c. ssDNA

    d. ssRNA

165. **The mode of transmission for IBR virus is:**

    a. Venereal

    b. Inhalation

    c. a and b

    d. None of these

166. The most effective chemical disinfectant to kill FMD virus is:

a. 2% formalin

b. 70% alcohol

c. 2% sodium hydroxide

d. 0.5% phenol

167. Hendra- and Nipah viruses belong to the family:

a. Paramyxoviridae

b. Orthomyxoviridae

c. Picornaviridae

d. Parvoviridae

168. Which are clinical manifestations of canine parvovirus infection?

a. Myocarditis

b. Haemorrhagic diarrhoea

c. Leukopenia

d. All of these

169. How many serotypes does bluetongue virus have?

a. 20

b. 24

c. 7

d. 9

170. Which is the wrong match?

a. Borrel bodies–Fowl pox

b. Guarneri bodies–smallpox

c. Negri bodies–rabies

d. All of these

171. Bovine diarrhoea virus belongs to the family:

a. Flaviviridae

b. Reoviridae

    c. Togaviridae

    d. Rhabdoviridae

172. Which of these is a viral triad?

    a. Rinderpest virus, measles virus and canine distemper virus

    b. Rinderpest virus, mumps virus and measles virus

    c. Measles, mumps and rubella viruses

    d. Rinderpest virus, reovirus and rhabdovirus

173. Bluetongue in sheep is caused by:

    a. Herpesvirus

    b. Birnavirus

    c. Picornavirus

    d. Orbivirus

174. Which virus has a reverse transcriptase enzyme?

    a. Retrovirus

    b. Reovirus

    c. Rabies virus

    d. Rotavirus

175. Which statement is not correct?

    a. Viruses multiply only in living cells

    b. Viral nucleic acid directs cell metabolism to synthesize viral components

    c. Viruses are not able to perform their own metabolic activities

    d. Viral genetic information resides only in DNA, not in RNA

176. Pseudorabies is caused by:

    a. Lyssavirus

    b. Picornavirus

    c. Paramyxovirus

    d. Herpesvirus

177. **Which disease of poultry is not caused by a virus?**

    a. Chronic respiratory disease

    b. Infectious bronchitis

    c. Fowl pox

    d. Ranikhet disease

178. **Infectious bronchitis is caused by:**

    a. Coronavirus

    b. Herpesvirus

    c. Picornavirus

    d. None of these

179. **A circulating monocyte can phagocytise:**

    a. Bacteria

    b. Viruses

    c. Ag-Ab complex

    d. All of these

180. **A dog bite wound should not be closed because:**

    a. The virus will be carried deeper

    b. Infection spreads quickly

    c. Bite wounds are contaminated

    d. All of these

181. **Bovine viral diarrhoea virus is antigenically related to:**

    a. Hog cholera and border disease

    b. PPR and measles

    c. CD and ND

    d. None of these

182. **Which type of Newcastle disease is most virulent:**

    a. Velogenic

    b. Mesogeni

c. Lentogenic

d. None of these

183. **Post-exposure prophylaxis for prevention of rabies is recommended for:**

a. 0, 3 and 7 days

b. 0, 3, 7, 14 and 28 days

c. 0 and 21 days

d. 0, 7, 21, 60 and 90 days

184. **Large eosinophilic intracytoplasmic inclusion bodies in fowl pox are known as:**

a. Bollinger bodies

b. Negri bodies

c. Guarneri bodies

d. Poschen bodies

185. **A 'brick-shape' is characteristic of:**

a. Birnavirus

b. Rabies virus

c. Poxvirus

d. All of these

186. **After entry into the peripheral nerves, the rabies virus travels at the rate of:**

a. 1–2 mm per hour

b. 1–2 cm per hour

c. 5–10 mm per hour

d. 5–10 cm per hour

187. **Which of the following diseases is caused by herpesvirus?**

a. IBR

b. Aujeszky's disease

c. MCF

d. All of these

188. **Contagious ecthyma is caused by a virus belonging to which family?**

   a. Picornaviridae

   b. Paramyxoviridae

   c. Orthomyxoviridae

   d. Poxviridae

189. **Capripoxvirus is composed of:**

   a. Goat pox virus

   b. Lumpy skin disease virus

   c. Sheep pox virus

   d. All of these

190. **The insect reported to be the biological vector of bluetongue virus is:**

   a. Mosquitoes

   b. Ticks

   c. Fleas

   d. Culicoides midges

191. **Maedi-visna (MV) in sheep is caused by:**

   a. Retrovirus

   b. Lyssavirus

   c. Picornavirus

   d. Paramyxovirus

192. **Pink eye is caused by Moraxella bovis and summer pink eye is caused by:**

   a. IBR virus

   b. CD virus

   c. Rabies virus

   d. None of these

193. **SMEDI in pigs is caused by:**

    a. Parvovirus

    b. Paramyxovirus

    c. PPR

    d. Coronavirus

194. **Jaagsiekte driving sickness in sheep is caused by:**

    a. Retrovirus

    b. Reovirus

    c. PPR virus

    d. Poxvirus

195. **Which virus has a unique double capsid?**

    a. Reovirus

    b. Retrovirus

    c. Picornavirus

    d. Paramyxovirus

196. **Canine parvovirus causes severe infection and death in young puppies due to the destruction of rapidly dividing cells in the:**

    a. Intestine

    b. Heart

    c. Bone marrow

    d. All of these

197. **Bullet-shaped negative-sense ssRNA virus is a characteristic feature in:**

    a. Ephemeral fever

    b. Rabies

    c. Vesicular stomatitis

    d. All of these

198. **Canine parvovirus replicates and destroys which highly dividing cells?**

    a. Intestinal cells

    b. Cardiac cells

    c. a and b

    d. None of these

199. **Multiplication of a virus in cytoplasm occurs in:**

    a. Papovaviridae

    b. Adenoviridae

    c. Herpesvirus

    d. Iridoviridae

200. **The genomic nucleic acid of the T-even phase is:**

    a. DNA

    b. r RNA

    c. RNA

    d. All of these

Answers

1.	d	30.	d	59.	a	88.	b
2.	a	31.	d	60.	c	89.	c
3.	c	32.	a	61.	a	90.	c
4.	c	33.	d	62.	d	91.	c
5.	c	34.	d	63.	c	92.	b
6.	a	35.	b	64.	c	93.	b
7.	a	36.	a	65.	b	94.	b
8.	b	37.	a	66.	c	95.	d
9.	c	38.	c	67.	d	96.	c
10.	b	39.	a	68.	c	97.	b
11.	d	40.	d	69.	b	98.	d
12.	a	41.	b	70.	c	99.	c
13.	a	42.	b	71.	c	100.	b
14.	b	43.	b	72.	b	101.	c
15.	b	44.	b	73.	b	102.	a
16.	d	45.	d	74.	d	103.	a
17.	b	46.	c	75.	a	104.	a
18.	a	47.	c	76.	b	105.	a
19.	a	48.	d	77.	c	106.	c
20.	d	49.	b	78.	c	107.	a
21.	a	50.	d	79.	c	108.	c
22.	d	51.	d	80.	b	109.	a
23.	b	52.	b	81.	b	110.	b
24.	b	53.	c	82.	a	111.	d
25.	c	54.	a	83.	d	112.	c
26.	b	55.	a	84.	d	113.	d
27.	a	56.	a	85.	d	114.	c
28.	a	57.	a	86.	d	115.	c
29.	c	58.	b	87.	d	116.	a

(Continued)

117.	b	138.	d	159.	b	180.	a
118.	a	139.	b	160.	c	181.	a
119.	a	140.	a	161.	b	182.	a
120.	c	141.	c	162.	c	183.	b
121.	a	142.	c	163.	a	184.	a
122.	b	143.	b	164.	d	185.	c
123.	d	144.	b	165.	b	186.	b
124.	a	145.	c	166.	c	187.	d
125.	c	146.	a	167.	a	188.	d
126.	b	147.	a	168.	d	189.	d
127.	b	148.	a	169.	b	190.	d
128.	d	149.	d	170.	d	191.	a
129.	c	150.	b	171.	a	192.	a
130.	a	151.	a	172.	a	193.	a
131.	c	152.	a	173.	d	194.	a
132.	c	153.	a	174.	a	195.	a
133.	c	154.	a	175.	d	196.	d
134.	c	155.	a	176.	a	197.	d
135.	d	156.	b	177.	a	198.	c
136.	b	157.	a	178.	a	199.	c
137.	c	158.	b	179.	d	200.	a

3 Bacterial Diseases

J.B. Kathiriya

Introduction

Veterinary bacteriology is a specialized branch of microbiology that deals with the study of bacteria, especially in relation to medicine and agriculture. The primary purpose of this chapter is to assist veterinarians and animal owners in providing optimal healthcare for animals by identifying those bacteria and fungi causing disease and by determining the antimicrobial agents to which the bacteria may respond *in vivo*. With continued research in the field of veterinary bacteriology, new concepts and findings have emerged and provide better understanding.

© CAB International 2024. *Key Questions in Preventative Farm Animal Medicine*
Volume 1: Types, Causes and Treatment of Infectious Diseases (ed. T. Rana)
DOI: 10.1079/9781800624726.0003

Multiple Choice Questions

1. **Bacteria can be characterised by:**

   a. Presence of mesosomes and absence of mitochondria

   b. Absence of mesosomes and presence of mitochondria

   c. Absence of both

   d. Presence of both

2. **The genetic material in bacteria is located in the:**

   a. Nucleus

   b. Nucleoid

   c. Cytoplasm

   d. Outer membrane

3. **Bacteria are named according to the:**

   a. Binomial system

   b. Trinomial system

   c. Polynomial system

   d. None of these

4. **Serum is sterilized by:**

   a. Autoclave

   b. Hot air oven

   c. Filtration

   d. Direct flaming

5. **Oil is sterilized by:**

   a. Incineration

   b. Hot air oven

   c. Filtration

   d. Tyndalization

6. **The molecules responsible for recognition of antigens by the immune system are:**

    a. B cell receptor

    b. T cell receptor

    c. MHC molecules

    d. All of these

7. **The antigen independent maturation of lymphoid cells occurs in the:**

    a. Primary lymphoid organ

    b. Secondary lymphoid organ

    c. Tertiary lymphoid organ

    d. None of these

8. **The antigen-dependent maturation of lymphoid cells occurs in the:**

    a. Primary lymphoid organ

    b. Secondary lymphoid organ

    c. Tertiary lymphoid organ

    d. None of these

9. **The predominant lymphocyte in blood circulation is:**

    a. B cell

    b. T cell

    c. a and b

    d. None of these

10. **Immunoglobulin is the surface receptor of:**

    a. B cells

    b. T cells

    c. a and b

    d. None of these

11. **Dark field microscopy is used to diagnose:**

   a. Listeriosis

   b. Leptospirosis

   c. Anthrax

   d. Q-fever

12. **A 'fried egg' colony appearance is seen in:**

   a. Histoplasma

   b. Mycoplasma

   c. Streptococci

   d. Pasturella

13. **Bottle-shaped cells and monopolar budding is seen in:**

   a. Malassezia

   b. Cryptococcus

   c. Histoplasma

   d. Candida

14. **CCPP is caused by:**

   a. *M. capricolum*

   b. *M. gallisepticum*

   c. *M. hyorhinis*

   d. *M. bovis*

15. **Bombblast growth in stab culture is seen in:**

   a. Streptococci

   b. Staphylococci

   c. Bacillus

   d. Listeria

16. **Nasal polyp is seen in:**

   a. Aspergillosis

   b. Rhinosporidiosis

c. Coccidiosis

d. Sporotrichosis

17. The Rose Bengal plate test is used for the diagnosis of:

a. Anthrax

b. Q-fever

c. Brucellosis

d. Coccidiosis

18. Which is an intracellular pathogen?

a. Brucella

b. Listeria

c. a and b

d. None of these

19. Avianhepatitis is caused by:

a. *P. multocida*

b. *C. jejuni*

c. *E. coli*

d. *S. pullorum*

20. Dimorhpic fungi are:

a. Blastomyces

b. Coccidioides

c. Histoplasmas

d. All of these

21. Spheroplasts are:

a. G-ve bacteria without a cell wall

b. G-ve bacteria with a partial cell wall

c. G-ve bacteria without a cytoplasmic membrane

d. G-ve bacteria with a partial cytoplasmic membrane

22. **Bacterial capsules:**

    a. Resist phagocytosis

    b. Prevent bacteriophage attachment

    c. Act as food reservoirs

    d. All of these

23. **Bacteria with flagella all over the surface are known as:**

    a. Amphitrichous

    b. Peritrichous

    c. Lopotrichous

    d. Atrichous

24. **Bacterial spores are resistant to:**

    a. Desiccation

    b. Disinfectant

    c. Radiation

    d. All of these

25. **Plasmids aid in:**

    a. Drug resistance

    b. Toxigenicity

    c. a and b

    d. None of these

26. **The antibody that mediates allergic reactions is:**

    a. IgG

    b. IgM

    c. IgE

    d. IgD

27. **The Fc region of IgG is formed by:**

    a. Heavy chain

    b. Light chain

c. Heavy and light chain

d. None of these

28.   The light chain is:

a. Kappa

b. Lambda

c. a and b

d. None of these

29.   The hinge region of IgG is rich in:

a. Proline, cysteine

b. Arginine

c. Methionine

d. None of these

30.   The changes in the amino acid sequences of the variable region of light and heavy chains are called:

a. Idiotypes

b. Isotypes

c. Allotypes

d. None of these

31.   Diamond skin disease is caused by:

a. *B. mallei*

b. *H. marasuis*

c. *E. rhusiopathiae*

d. *Y. enterocolitica*

32.   A malignant carbuncle is a cutaneous form of:

a. Anthrax

b. Q fever

c. Brucellosis

d. Coccidiosis

33. **A Nagler's reaction is characteristic of:**

    a. *C. tetani*

    b. *C. septicum*

    c. *C. haemolyticum*

    d. *C. perfringens*

34. **A Hotis test is used to diagnose:**

    a. Anthrax

    b. Q fever

    c. Brucellosis

    d. Mastitis

35. **Edwards media is used in the isolation of:**

    a. Staphylococci

    b. Leptospira

    c. Bacillus

    d. Streptococci

36. **Aseptic technique was developed by:**

    a. E. Jenner

    b. J. Lister

    c. R. Koch

    d. L. Pasteur

37. **The term vaccine was coined by:**

    a. E. Jenner

    b. J. Tyndall

    c. R. Koch

    d. L. Pasteur

38. **The chemical basis of specificity of immune reaction and blood groups in humans was discovered by:**

    a. E. Metchnikoff

    b. R. Koch

c. K. Landsteiner

d. F. Hesse

39. The complement system was discovered by:

a. E. Metchnikoff

b. J. Bordet

c. K. Landsteiner

d. L. Pasteur

40. Who is known as the 'father of bacteriology'?

a. E. Jenner

b. J. Lister

c. R. Koch

d. L. Pasteur

41. The electron microscope was invented by:

a. Wright brothers

b. Ruska and Mortom

c. Rousand Border

d. L. Pasteur

42. The resolution limit of an ordinary microscope is:

a. 200 nm

b. 250 µm

c. 200 µm

d. 400 nm

43. The shortest distance by which two particles are separated to give distinct images is known as:

a. Magnification

b. Numerical aperture

c. Resolving power

d. None of these

44. The three principles on which the compound microscope works are magnification, resolving power and:

    a. Illusion

    b. Numerical aperture

    c. Illumination

    d. Wavelength

45. The ribosome system in bacteria is:

    a. 70 S

    b. 75 S

    c. 80 S

    d. 85 S

46. The major surface receptor of a natural killer cell is:

    a. CD4

    b. CD8

    c. CD56

    d. None of these

47. The glycoproteins produced by virus infected cells are called:

    a. Interleukins

    b. Interferons

    c. Antigens

    d. Leukotrines

48. Acute phase proteins are:

    a. Lectins

    b. Fibronectins

    c. Iron binding proteins

    d. All of these

49. **The sentinel cells are:**

   a. Macrophages

   b. Dendritic cells

   c. Mast cells

   d. All of these

50. **The B lymphocytes of birds mature in:**

   a. Bone marrow

   b. Bursa of fabricious

   c. Spleen

   d. Blood

51. **T lymphocytes mature in:**

   a. Bone marrow

   b. Thymus

   c. Spleen

   d. Blood

52. **Sentinel cells recognize pathogens by:**

   a. TLR

   b. NLR

   c. a and b

   d. None of these

53. **T cells recognize:**

   a. Antigen alone

   b. Antigen in association with MHC–II only

   c. Both a and b

   d. None

54. **T cells recognize antigens through:**

   a. TCR

   b. TCR-CD3 complex

c. BCR

d. None of these

55.   Cells bearing CD4 recognize:

a. MHC–I

b. MHC–II

c. MHC–III

d. All of these

56.   An Anton test is performed to establish:

a. Listeria

b. Yersinia

c. a and b

d. None of these

57.   Polymyxin is produced by:

a. *C .polymyxa*

b. *B. polymyxa*

c. *B. subtilis*

d. *C. perfringens*

58.   Lemon-shaped bacilli are seen in:

a. *C. chuvoei*

b. *C. tetani*

c. *C. perfringens*

d. *C. colinum*

59.   Ray fungus is the common name for:

a. *A. fumigatus*

b. *M. canis*

c. *A. bovis*

d. *T. rubrum*

60. **Anthrax spores are effectively killed by:**

    a. 4% KMNO4

    b. 4% phenol

    c. 4% NaOH

    d. None of these

61. **Strauss test in male guinea pigs can be used for the detection of the following bacteria except:**

    a. *B. mallei*

    b. *A. lignieresii*

    c. *B. abortus*

    d. *P. multocida*

62. **The IMViC test for *E.coli* is:**

    a. ++ --

    b. + ---

    c. +- +-

    d. -- ++

63. **Tumbling motility is seen in:**

    a. Listeria

    b. Leptospira

    c. Bacillus

    d. Clostridia

64. **The kitten test is done to diagnose:**

    a. Streptococci

    b. Staphylococci

    c. Bacillus

    d. Listeria

65. **Serotyping of *E. coli* is based on the antigen extracted from:**

    a. Somatic

    b. Capsule

c. Flagella

d. All of these

66. **Members of the order Mononnegavirales include:**

a. Rhabdoviridae

b. Picornaviridae

c. Birnaviridae

d. Coronavirdae

67. **The order Nidovirales comprises:**

a. Coronavirdae

b. Arterivirdae

c. Both a and b

d. None of these

68. **Streaks of haemorrhage are seen in the large intestine in animals affected with:**

a. Rinderpest

b. PPR

c. a and b

d. None of these

69. **The first step in viral replication is:**

a. Attachment

b. Uncoating

c. Replication of nucleic acid

d. Release

70. **The polymerase enzyme functions as:**

a. Transcriptase

b. Replicase

c. a and b

d. None of these

71. **The S19 vaccine is used in:**

    a. Brucellosis

    b. Leptospirosis

    c. Anthrax

    d. Q fever

72. **The mycobacterium affecting armadillos and chimpanzees is:**

    a. *M. tuberculosis*

    b. *M. leprae*

    c. *M. africanum*

    d. *M. microti*

73. **Glassers disease in pigs is caused by:**

    a. *B. mallei*

    b. *H. parasuis*

    c. *E. rhusiopathiae*

    d. *Y. enterocolitica*

74. **Romanowsky staining is used to detect:**

    a. Haemobartonella

    b. Mycobacterium

    c. Leptospira

    d. Trichophyton

75. **Lateral bodies are present in the structures of:**

    a. Vacciniavirus

    b. Cow pox virus

    c. Variolavirus

    d. All of these

76. **The lumpy skin disease is a form of:**

    a. Leporipoxvirus

    b. Orthopoxvirus

c. Suipoxvirus

d. Capripoxvirus

77. **Phylogenetically, the sheep pox and goat pox viruses are**

a. Identical

b. Distinct

c. a and b

d. None of these

78. **Sheep pox produces inclusion bodies which are:**

a. Intranuclear basophilic

b. Intracytoplasmic basophilic

c. Intranuclear acidophilic

d. Intracytoplasmic acidophilic

79. **Previously, African swine fever virus was classed as part of which family?**

a. Poxviridae

b. Herpesviridae

c. Adenoviridae

d. Iridovirdae

80. **African swine fever virus is maintained in the life cycle of:**

a. Ornithodorus

b. Rhipicephalus

c. a and b

d. None of these

81. **Parvovirus multiplies only in the nuclei of:**

a. Resting cells

b. Dividing cells

c. a and b

d. None of these

82. **Feline panleukopenia virus belongs to:**

a. Parvoviridae

b. Circoviridae

c. Adenoviridae

d. Caliciviridae

83. **Porcine parvovirus is a major cause of:**

a. Stillbirth

b. Mummified fetus

c. EED, infertility

d. All of these

84. **Chicken anaemia virus belongs to:**

a. Caliciviridae

b. Circoviridae

c. Herpesviridae

d. Parvoviridae

85. **Post-weaning multisystemic wasting syndrome is caused by:**

a. Porcine circovirus-2

b. Porcine circovirus-5

c. Vesicular exanthema

d. None of these

86. **Short, hair-like projections for attachment and genetic trans-fer in bacteria include:**

a. Flagella

b. Fimbria

c. Plasmid

d. All of these

87. **The autonomously replicating extra-chromosomal double stranded DNA molecule present in bacteria is called:**

    a. Plasmid

    b. Episome

    c. Phage

    d. Transposon

88. **Agar is a source of carbohydrate for:**

    a. Most bacteria

    b. Only a few bacteria

    c. None of the bacteria

    d. All bacteria

89. **The acquisition of the DNA molecule by bacterial cells from the environment is called:**

    a. Transformation

    b. Transduction

    c. Conjugation

    d. None of these

90. **Bacteria that grow at 50–60 °C are known as:**

    a. Psychrophiles

    b. Mesophiles

    c. Thermophiles

    d. Halophiles

91. **The ability of a cell to acquire DNA from the environment is called:**

    a. Competence

    b. Compatibility

    c. Interference

    d. None of these

92. **The first bacterial genome to be sequenced was:**

    a. *Salmonella typimurium*

    b. *Bacillus anthracis*

    c. *Pseudomonas aeruginosa*

    d. *Haemophilus influenza*

93. **Which acid-producing bacteria converts lactose into lactic acid in milk?**

    a. *Streptococcus cremoris*

    b. *Staphylococcus aureus*

    c. *Bacillus cereus*

    d. *Clostridium botulinm*

94. **The most common bacterium causing joint pain is:**

    a. *Brucella*

    b. *Shigella*

    c. *Salmonella*

    d. *Clostridia*

95. **Galacto toxins in milk are produced by:**

    a. *Streptococci* spp.

    b. Contact of milk with a steel vessel

    c. Contact of milk with a copper vessel

    d. *Serratia* spp.

96. **Which agent is used against anaerobic bacteria as well as protozoa?**

    a. Mebendazole

    b. Metronidazole

    c. Methicillin

    d. Marbofloxacin

97. **Streptococcus is characterized by:**

    a. Gram-positive cocci

    b. Catalase-ve

    c. Arranged in chain

    d. All of these

98. **Cold enrichment is required for the isolation of:**

    a. *Listeria monocytogenes*

    b. *Staph. aureus*

    c. *Erysipelothrix*

    d. *Clostridium tetani*

99. **Which bacteria are responsible for food poisoning?**

    a. *Staph. aureus*

    b. *Bacillus cereus*

    c. *Clostridium botulinum*

    d. All of these

100. **A dysgonic species of mycobacterium is:**

    a. *M. bovis*

    b. *M. avium*

    c. *M. tuberculosis*

    d. *M. phlei*

101. **Satellite growth on blood agar plates in the presence of *Staph. aureus* is characteristic of:**

    a. *Pasteurella*

    b. *Haemophillus*

    c. *Actinobacillus*

    d. *Mycoplasma*

102. **The di-deoxy chain termination method of DNA sequencing is called the:**

    a. Maxam-Gilbert method

    b. Sanger method

    c. Pyrosequencing method

    d. Nanopore sequencing method

103. **The pH of TRIS-saturated phenol used for the purpose of DNA isolation should be:**

    a. 5.0

    b. 6.0

    c. 7.0

    d. 8.0

104. **A DNA molecule as big as 10 MB can be separated by:**

    a. Polyacrylamide gel electrophoresis

    b. Agrose gel electrophoresis

    c. Pulse field electrophoresis

    d. None of these

105. **The blotting technique used for the detection of DNA molecules is known as:**

    a. Southern blot

    b. Northern blot

    c. Western blot

    d. Eastern blot

106. **The blotting technique used for the detection of RNA molecules is known as:**

    a. Southern blot

    b. Northern blot

    c. Western blot

    d. Eastern blot

107. **The blotting technique used for the detection of protein is known as:**

   a. Southern blot

   b. Northern blot

   c. Western blot

   d. Eastern blot

108. **In southern blot, the labelled nucleic acid used to detect complementary sequences is called:**

   a. Template

   b. Primer

   c. Probe

   d. None of these

109. **Crop mycosis in poultry is caused by:**

   a. Bacteria

   b. Mycoplasma

   c. Fungi

   d. Viruses

110. **Brooder's pneumonia in poultry is caused by:**

   a. *Candida albicans*

   b. *Aspergillus fumigatus*

   c. *Haemophilus paragallinarum*

   d. *Pasturella multocida*

111. **Which bacteria require a living medium for their growth?**

   a. Mycoplasma and leptospira

   b. Chlamydia and rickettsia

   c. Rickettsia and mycoplasma

   d. None of these

112. A palisade arrangement is characteristic of:

a. Corynebacterium

b. *E. coli*

c. Campylobacter

d. Listeria

113. Mycoplasma organisms are pleomorphic due to:

a. Absence of a rigid plasma membrane

b. Absence of a rigid cell wall

c. Their small size

d. All of these

114. Periodic ophthalmia in horses is a sequel of:

a. Glanders

b. Mycoplasmosis

c. Equine leptospirosis

d. Babesiosis

115. Chlamydia can be stained with the following stains except:

a. Gram stain

b. Macchiavello stain

c. Gimenez stain

d. Castaneda stain

116. A tuberculin test is based on:

a. Delayed hypersensitivity

b. Arthus reaction

c. Anaphylactic reaction

d. All of these

117. Calf hood vaccination is advisable for

a. Brucellosis

b. Salmonellosis

c. Pasteurellosis

d. Neonatal calf diarrhoea

118. **Germ tube production is characteristic of:**

a. *Candida albicans*

b. *Corynebacterium pyogenes*

c. *Cryptococcus neoformans*

d. *Pseudomonas aeruginosa*

119. **Experimentally, *Mycobacterium leprae* can be cultivated on:**

a. Bacterial media with mycobactin

b. Cell culture system

c. 9-banded armadillo

d. None of these

120. **For transformation reactions competent *E. coli* cells can be prepared by treating log phase *E. coli* cells with:**

a. Calcium chloride

b. Magnesium chloride

c. EDTA

d. None of these

121. **A DNA molecule from an external source can be inserted into host cells by:**

a. Heat shock treatment

b. Electroporation

c. Lipofection

d. None of these

122. **In a PCR reaction, the use of two short oligonucleotides flanking the DNA sequence to be amplified is called:**

a. Primer

b. Probe

c. Template

d. None of these

123. **The source of the Taq polymerase used in the PCR reaction is:**

a. *E. coli*

b. Thermusaquaticus

c. a and b

d. None of these

124. **The source of the 'reverse transcriptase enzyme' used for cDNA synthesis is:**

a. Moloney murine leukaemia virus (MuLV)

b. Avian myeloblastosis virus (AMV)

c. a and b

d. None of these

125. **Quantitative studies using PCR technique can be done with:**

a. RT-PCR

b. Real-time PCR

c. Micro array

d. None of these

126. **Most type II restriction endonucleases recognize and cleave to DNA within a particular sequence of 4–8 nucleotides, which have twofold rotational symmetry. Such sequences are called:**

a. Palindromes

b. Short tandem repeats

c. a and b

d. None of these

127. **For restriction analysis of a DNA molecule, the type of re-striction endonucleases used are called:**

a. Type I RE

b. Type II RE

c. Type III RE

d. None of these

128. **The chief source of leptospira is:**

   a. Blood

   b. Urine

   c. Milk

   d. Faeces

129. **Growth of brucella organisms is favoured due to:**

   a. Erythritol

   b. Sorbitol

   c. Glucose

   d. Protein

130. ***E. coli*:**

   a. Grows at 15-40 °C

   b. Is a lactose fermenter

   c. Is motile

   d. All of these

131. **Spore-forming bacteria include:**

   a. *Bacillus*

   b. *Clostridium*

   c. a and b

   d. None of these

132. **Isoschizomers are restriction enzymes which:**

   a. Recognize and cut the same sequence

   b. Recognize the same sequence but the cut site varies

   c. a and b

   d. None of these

133. **Neoschizomers are restriction enzymes which:**

   a. Recognize and cut the same sequence

   b. Recognize the same sequence but the cut site varies

c. a and b

d. None of these

134. Which enzyme is used to join two DNA molecules?

a. DNA gyrase

b. DNA ligase

c. Topoisomerase

d. Helicase

135. Which of the following has the highest density?

a. Relaxed genomic DNA

b. Supercoiled DNA

c. Plasmid

d. RNA

136. A homopolymer tail can be added by using the enzyme:

a. Ligase

b. Phosphate kinase

c. Terminal deoxytransferase

d. None of these

137. The plasmids maintained in host cells in multiple copies are called:

a. Relaxed

b. Stringent

c. Conjugative

d. None of these

138. The plasmids maintained in host cells in a limited number of copies are called:

a. Relaxed

b. Stringent

c. Conjugative

d. None

139. **What is the name for RNA that catalyses biological reactions, such as self-splicing introns?**

    a. Enzyme

    b. Ribozyme

    c. Sliceosome

    d. None of these

140. **The 2 μm plasmid is found in:**

    a. *Escherichia coli*

    b. *Pneumococcus*

    c. *Bacillus anthracis*

    d. *Saccharomyces Cerevisiae*

141. **Which of the following statements is true for the life cycle of lysogenic phages:**

    a. They immediately induce lysis of host cells for the release of new virions

    b. Phage DNA is integrated with the host DNA and retained for several generations

    c. Both a and b depending on environmental conditions

    d. None of these

142. **Genes cloned with M13-based vectors can be obtained in the form of:**

    a. Single stranded DNA

    b. Double stranded DNA

    c. Single stranded RNA

    d. None of these

143. **At 600 nm, one unit optical density (OD) of *E. coli* culture corresponds roughly to:**

    a. 1 X 106 cells/ml

    b. 1 X 107 cells/ml

    c. 1 X 108 cells/ml

    d. 1 X 109 cells/ml

144. **EDTA present in lysis solution has which functions?**

   a. Chelates Mg++ ions and thus inhibits activity of enzyme DNase

   b. Removes Mg++ ions that are essential for preserving the overall structure of the cell envelope

   c. a and b

   d. None of these

145. **Which of the following matches is incorrect?**

   a. SDS–cell lysis

   b. EDTA–chelating Mg++ ions

   c. Proteinase K–degradation of protein

   d. Isoamyl alcohol–precipitation of DNA

146. **CTAB used during DNA isolation, forms complexes with:**

   a. Lipids

   b. Proteins

   c. Carbohydrates

   d. None of these

147. **Guanidinium thiocynate is useful in DNA isolation because:**

   a. It forms complexes with DNA molecules

   b. It denatures and dissolves all biochemical substances other than nucleic acid

   c. DNA binds tightly to silica particles in its presence

   d. b and c

148. **The bacterial name for venereal disease is:**

   a. Brucellosis

   b. Campylobacteriosis

   c. Genital tuberculosis

   d. Leptospirosis

149. **A component of egg white having antibacterial activity is:**

    a. Lysozyme

    b. Avidine

    c. Transferine

    d. All of these

150. **The process by which zoonotic diseases are perpetuated in nature by a single vertebrate species is known as:**

    a. Cyclozoonosis

    b. Direct zoonosis

    c. Metazoonosis

    d. Amphizoonosis

151. **Which of these is a form of bacterial zoonosis?**

    a. Brucellosis

    b. Leptospirosis

    c. Listeriosis

    d. All of these

152. **Yellow fever is transmitted by.**

    a. Aedes aegypti

    b. Argus

    c. Ioxides

    d. Simules

153. **An outbreak of disease in a bird population is termed as:**

    a. Epizootic

    b. Epidemic

    c. Epornitics

    d. All of these

154. **Corynebacteria can be characterized as:**

    a. Nonmotile, nonsporing, aerobic, gram-positive bacilli

    b. Motile, nonsporing, aerobic, gram-positive bacilli

c. Motile, sporing, aerobic, gram-positive bacilli

d. Nonmotile, sporing, anaerobic, gram-positive bacilli

155. **The cells parasitized in host by Rickettsia are:**

a. Erythrocytes

b. Vascular endothelial cells

c. Neutrophils

d. Monocytes

156. **Dimorphic fungi produces:**

a. Mould-type growth at 370 °C

b. Yeast-type growth at 220 °C

c. Mould-type growth at 370 °C and yeast-type growth at 220 °C.

d. Yeast-type growth at 370 °C and mould type growth at 220 °C

157. **The organism present in high concentrations of pigeon droppings is:**

a. *Candida albicans*

b. *Cryptococcus neoformans*

c. *Rhinosporidium seeberi*

d. *Aspergillus flavus*

158. **Which of the following is an incorrect match?**

a. Diene's stain–mycoplasma

b. Fontana stain–spirochaetes

c. Machiavello stain–chlamydia

d. Acid fast stain–staphylococci

159. **A Strauss reaction is positive for:**

a. *Brucella abortus*

b. *Pseudomonas mallei*

c. *Actinobacillus lignieresii*

d. All of these

160. **The Weil-Felix test is an agglutination reaction between:**

    a. Antibody against Rickettsia and antigen from Pseudomonas

    b. Antibody against Rickettsia and antigen from Staphylococci

    c. Antibody against Rickettsia and antigen from Brucella.

    d. Antibody against Rickettsia and antigen from Proteus

161. **IMViC pattern of salmonella is:**

    a. $+ + - -$

    b. $+ - + -$

    c. $- - + +$

    d. $- + - +$

162. **Which of the following showing buoyant density of DNA, RNA and protein is correct:**

    a. RNA>DNA>protein

    b. Protein>RNA>DNA

    c. DNA>RNA>protein

    d. Protein>DNA>RNA

163. **Intercalation of ethidium bromide (etBr) in a DNA molecule will:**

    a. Increase the buoyant density of the molecule

    b. Decrease the buoyant density of the molecule

    c. Does not affect the buoyant density of the molecule

    d. None of these

164. **Exonucleases:**

    a. Remove nucleotides one at a time from the end of a DNA molecule

    b. Break internal phospho-diester bonds within a DNA molecule

    c. Remove nucleotides only in 3'–5' direction

    d. Remove nucleotides only in 5'–3' direction

165. **Endonucleases:**

   a. Remove nts one at a time from the end of a DNA molecule

   b. Break internal phospho-diester bonds within a DNA molecule

   c. Remove nts only in 3'–5' direction

   d. Remove nts only in 5'–3' direction

166. **The enzyme used to remove the phosphate group at the 5' end of a DNA molecule is:**

   a. Alkaline phosphatase

   b. Polynucleotide kinase

   c. Terminal deoxytransferase

   d. Topoisomerase

167. **The enzyme used to add the phosphate group at the free 5' end of a DNA molecule is:**

   a. Alkaline phosphatase

   b. Polynucleotide kinase

   c. Terminal deoxytransferase

   d. Topoisomerase

168. **The enzyme that changes the conformation of covalently closed circular DNA by introducing or removing supercoils is:**

   a. Alkaline phosphatase

   b. Polynucleotide kinase

   c. Terminal deoxy transferase

   d. Topoisomerase

169. **Eco RI produces:**

   a. Blunt end

   b. Sticky end

   c. a and b

   d. None of these

170. **The specific position on a DNA molecule where DNA replication begins is called:**

    a. Replication fork

    b. Origin of replication

    c. Start point of replication

    d. None of these

171. **The primary culture medium to grow fungi is:**

    a. L.J. medium

    b. NA

    c. SDA

    d. Trypticase soy agar

172. **The following are motile except :**

    a. *Cl. septicum*

    b. *Cl. welchii*

    c. *Cl. botulinum*

    d. *Cl. tetani*

173. **Which medium does not transmit leptospirae?**

    a. Contaminated food and water

    b. Broken skin

    c. Mucous membranes

    d. Ticks and mites

174. **Which does not give an acid-fast reaction?**

    a. Mycobacterium

    b. Nocardia

    c. Rhodococcus

    d. Leptospira

175. **Which area does *E. coli* share with *Klebsiella*?**

    a. Motility

    b. Mucoid colonies

c. IMViC test

d. Lactose fermentation

176.   A Strauss test is positive except in:

a. *Br. abortus*

b. *Actinobacillus lignieresii*

c. *Past. multocida*

d. *Burkholderia mallei*

177.   Which are examples of differential staining methods?

a. Gram method

b. Acid fast method

c. a and b

d. None of these

178.   A type of connective tissue cell that produces and secretes histamine is:

a. Plasma cell

b. T TH cell

c. Mast cell

d. Neutrophil

179.   Which is a serum containing induced antibodies?

a. Antiserum

b. Immune serum

c. Hyperimmune serum

d. All of these

180.   Which is an organ of immunity in birds?

a. Bursa of fabricius

b. Cloaca

c. Proventriculus

d. Air sacs

181. **Certain spirochetes are observed by:**

    a. Telescopic technique

    b. Ultraviolet microscopy

    c. Dark field microscopy

    d. None of these

182. **Marek's disease is isolated in a diseased bird using:**

    a. Feather follicle

    b. Liner

    c. Nerve trunk

    d. Eye secretion

183. **Which of these consists of SS plus stand linear RNA?**

    a. Picorneviridae

    b. Parvoviridae

    c. Paramyzoviridae

    d. Reoviridae

184. **Which of the following is an oncogene?**

    a. gag

    b. pol

    c. em

    d. sre

185. **The genus *Thogotovirus* belongs to the family**

    a. Orthomyxoviridae

    b. Paramyxoviridae

    c. Rhabdoviridae

    d. Ciroviridae

186. **Which of the following organisms gain access to the bovine udder during milking?**

    a. *Staphylococcus aureus*

    b. *E. coli*

c. *Pseudomonas* spp.

d. *Klebsiella* spp.

187.   **Miasmatic theory was proposed by:**

a. Themisson

b. Girolamo Frocaistoro

c. Thassalus

d. Hippocrates

188.   **Contagion theory was proposed by:**

a. Girolamo Frocaistro

b. Antonie van Leeuwenhoek

c. Athanisius Kircher

d. Francesco Redi

189.   **Louis Pasteur developed vaccines against the following diseases except:**

a. Anthrax

b. Fowl cholera

c. Tuberculosis

d. Rabies

190.   **The first person to use a solid medium for cultivating bacteria was:**

a. Louis Pasteur

b. Francesco Redi

c. Robert Koch

d. Theodor Schwann

191.   **Cork-screw shaped form of bacteria are:**

a. Spirochetes

b. Bacilli

c. Actinomycetes

d. Stalked bacteria

192. Organisms lacking a rigid cell wall are included under:

a. Gracilicutes

b. Firmicutes

c. Mendosicutes

d. Tenericutes

193. A gram-positive bacterial cell wall, in addition to peptidoglycan contain:

a. Mycolic acid

b. Teichioc acid

c. Muramic acid

d. Pimilic acid

194. The linkage between N-acetylglucosamine and N-acetylmuramic acid is:

a. Beta 1, 4

b. Beta 1, 3

c. Beta 1, 2

d. Beta 1, 5

195. The capsule and slime layers are together known as:

a. Endoplasmin

b. Glycocalyx

c. Exotoxin

d. Somatic antigen

196. Which type of flagella arrangement is seen in *Pseudomonas aeruginosa*?

a. Peritrichous

b. Amphitrichous

c. Lophotrichous

d. Monotrichous

197. **Which among the cocci organisms have flagella?**

    a. Sporocercina

    b. Rhodococcus

    c. Planococcus

    d. All these

198. **Impermeability of spore is due to:**

    a. Poly-D-glutamic acid

    b. Calcium dipicolinic acid

    c. Thecoic acid

    d. Diaminopimelic acid

199. **Which among the following is a diplococci?**

    a. Micrococci

    b. Neisseria

    c. Streptococci

    d. Rhodococci

200. **Feulgen staining is used to stain _____ which appears _____ in colour:**

    a. Nucleoid, purple

    b. Cytoplasm, blue

    c. Ribosome, purple

    d. Volutin granules, red

201. **Cooked meat media can be used in which cultures?**

    a. Anaerobic

    b. Capnophilic

    c. Mesophilic

    d. Thermophilic

202. **The method used to preserve bacteria in powder form is:**

    a. Tyndallization

    b. Lyophilization

c. Deep freezing

d. Cryopreservation

203. **The refractive index of Canada balsam is:**

a. 1.535

b. 1.524

c. 1.483

d. 1.460

204. **Which of the following group of bacteria is considered as a link between bacteria and virus?**

a. Actinomycetes

b. Spirochetes

c. Mycoplasmas

d. Vibrios

205. **Fractional sterilization was devised by:**

a. L. Pasteur

b. John Tyndall

c. John Snow

d. Joseph Lister

206. **A Seitz filter is used for filtering:**

a. Culture broth

b. Serum

c. Toxins from culture

d. Viral growth medium

207. **The preservative used for serum is:**

a. Merthiolate

b. HCHO

c. 70% alcohol

d. 10% alcohol

208. A Garrod test is used:

   a. To evaluate virulence of bacteria

   b. To check the phenol coefficient

   c. To check antibiotic susceptibility

   d. To estimate D-value

209. Anaerobes cannot withstand oxygen due to lack of:

   a. Superoxide dismutase

   b. Catalase

   c. Peroxidase

   d. a and b

210. Piezophiles are bacteria which can withstand great:

   a. Atmospheric pressure

   b. Osmotic pressure

   c. Radiation

   d. Temperature

211. The ratio of the diameter of an objective lens to its focal length is called:

   a. Numerical aperture

   b. Resolution

   c. Magnification

   d. None of these

212. Which are examples of positive eye pieces?

   a. Huygenian eyepieces

   b. Ramsden eyepieces

   c. a and b

   d. None of these

213. **Which type of microscopy is used to determine the dry mass of living cells and their nuclei?**

    a. Darkfield microscopy

    b. Laser microscopy

    c. Interference microscopy

    d. Fluorescence microscopy

214. **Which specimen type must be used in electron microscopy?**

    a. Hydrated

    b. Dehydrated

    c. Thick

    d. Stained

215. **Which among the following contain sterol in the cytoplasmic membrane?**

    a. Spirochetes

    b. Mycoplasma

    c. Chlamydia

    d. Clostridia

216. **What are also known as PPLO?**

    a. Rickettsiae

    b. Mycoplasma

    c. Mycobacteria

    d. Chlamydia

217. **What produces packets of 8 organisms or multiples of 8?**

    a. Neisseria

    b. Sarcina

    c. Veillonella

    d. All of these

218. **A normal 'fir tree' appearance in a gelatine stab medium is produced by:**

    a. *Bacillus anthracis*

    b. *Clostridium*

    c. *Erysipelothrix*

    d. *Salmonella*

219. **The primary stain in gram staining is:**

    a. Crystal violet

    b. Methylene blue

    c. Safranin

    d. Carbolfuchsin

220. **In the Hucker staining method, gram positive cells appear as what colour?**

    a. Blue

    b. Pink

    c. Violet

    d. Dark red

221. **Which among the following is incorrect concerning the negative staining of bacteria?**

    a. Used to study cell shape

    b. Can be done with eosin or nigrosin

    c. Stain does not penetrate the cell

    d. Heat fixation is required

222. **Which among the following is acid-fast positive?**

    a. Mycoplasma

    b. Nocardia

    c. Neisseria

    d. Fusobacterium

223. **The *Truant* staining fluorescence method is used for:**

a. Endoscopy

b. Acid fast bacteria

c. Flagella

d. Gram-positive bacteria

224. **A popping test is performed in the staining of:**

a. Exospores

b. Endospores

c. Pili

d. Flagella

225. **Which is used for endospore staining?**

a. Schaeffer-Fulton staining

b. Donner staining

c. Burke staining

d. a and b

226. **Which is used for flagellar staining?**

a. Gray staining

b. Leyson staining

c. Dorner staining

d. a and b

227. **Which is used in an Ames test?**

a. *Salmonella typhimurium*

b. *Shigella dysentriae*

c. *Staphylococcus aureus*

d. *Sreptococcus pneumoniae*

228. **Muller Hinton agar is used in:**

a. Ames test

b. Replica plating method

c. Antibiotic sensitivity test

d. Penicillin enrichment of mutants

229. **Calcium chloride-treated bacterial cells are competent for:**

a. Transduction

b. Transformation

c. Plasmid replication

d. Conjugation

230. **The indicator in urea broth medium is:**

a. Phenol red

b. Bromocresol purple

c. Methyl red

d. Bromothymol blue

231. **The IMViC reaction for Yersinia is:**

a. $+ + - -$

b. $- + - +$

c. $- - + +$

d. $- + - -$

232. **Indole production can be detected by:**

a. Barritt's reagent

b. Kovac's reagent

c. Collin's reagent

d. Baeyer's reagent

233. **Which shows mixed acid fermentation of glucose?**

a. Shigella

b. Klebsiella

c. Enterobacter

d. Serratia

234. **Which formulation is used as a cryoprotectant in the storage of bacterial cultures at -700 °C?**

    a. 10% glycerol

    b. 10% DMSO

    c. 15% glycerol

    d. 15% DMSO

235. **A Vogesproskeur test is based on the ability of an organism to produce what in glucose phosphate broth?**

    a. Urea

    b. Pyruvic acid

    c. Acetoin

    d. Phenylenediamine

Answers

1.	a	**32.**	a	**63.**	a	**94.**	a
2.	b	**33.**	d	**64.**	b	**95.**	c
3.	a	**34.**	d	**65.**	d	**96.**	b
4.	c	**35.**	d	**66.**	a	**97.**	d
5.	b	**36.**	b	**67.**	c	**98.**	a
6.	a	**37.**	d	**68.**	b	**99.**	d
7.	b	**38.**	c	**69.**	a	**100.**	a
8.	a	**39.**	b	**70.**	c	**101.**	a
9.	c	**40.**	c	**71.**	a	**102.**	b
10.	b	**41.**	b	**72.**	b	**103.**	d
11.	b	**42.**	a	**73.**	b	**104.**	c
12.	b	**43.**	c	**74.**	a	**105.**	a
13.	a	**44.**	c	**75.**	d	**106.**	b
14.	a	**45.**	a	**76.**	d	**107.**	c
15.	d	**46.**	c	**77.**	b	**108.**	a
16.	b	**47.**	b	**78.**	d	**109.**	c
17.	a	**48.**	d	**79.**	d	**110.**	b
18.	c	**49.**	d	**80.**	a	**111.**	b
19.	b	**50.**	b	**81.**	b	**112.**	a
20.	d	**51.**	b	**82.**	a	**113.**	b
21.	b	**52.**	c	**83.**	d	**114.**	c
22.	d	**53.**	b	**84.**	b	**115.**	a
23.	b	**54.**	b	**85.**	a	**116.**	a
24.	d	**55.**	b	**86.**	a	**117.**	a
25.	c	**56.**	d	**87.**	d	**118.**	a
26.	c	**57.**	a	**88.**	c	**119.**	c
27.	c	**58.**	b	**89.**	a	**120.**	a
28.	c	**59.**	b	**90.**	c	**121.**	d
29.	a	**60.**	a	**91.**	a	**122.**	a
30.	a	**61.**	a	**92.**	d	**123.**	b
31.	c	**62.**	a	**93.**	a	**124.**	c

(Continued)

125.	b	153.	c	181.	c	209.	d
126.	a	154.	a	182.	a	210.	a
127.	d	155.	b	183.	a	211.	a
128.	b	156.	d	184.	d	212.	b
129.	d	157.	b	185.	a	213.	c
130.	c	158.	d	186.	a	214.	b
131.	a	159.	d	187.	d	215.	b
132.	b	160.	d	188.	a	216.	b
133.	b	161.	d	189.	c	217.	b
134.	d	162.	a	190.	c	218.	b
135.	c	163.	b	191.	a	219.	a
136.	a	164.	a	192.	d	220.	c
137.	b	165.	b	193.	b	221.	d
138.	b	166.	a	194.	a	222.	b
139.	d	167.	b	195.	b	223.	b
140.	b	168.	d	196.	c	224.	b
141.	a	169.	b	197.	d	225.	d
142.	d	170.	b	198.	b	226.	d
143.	c	171.	c	199.	b	227.	a
144.	d	172.	b	200.	a	228.	c
145.	a	173.	d	201.	a	229.	b
146.	d	174.	d	202.	b	230.	a
147.	b	175.	d	203.	a	231.	d
148.	b	176.	c	204.	c	232.	b
149.	a	177.	c	205.	b	233.	a
150.	b	178.	c	206.	b	234.	a
151.	a	179.	d	207.	a	235.	c
152.	c	180.	a	208.	b		

4 Fungal Diseases

J. Jyothi and M. Bhavya Sree

Introduction

Fungal diseases are important, since they affect the health and productivity of animals. Some cause complete cessation of milk yield or abortion while others cause superficial infections that can affect the fur and the quality of the hide. These diseases also have zoonotic importance.

Fungi constitute a large heterogenous group of organisms ranging from unicellular yeast bodies like cryptococcus to more common mycelium-forming types such as aspergillus.

Multiple Choice Questions

1. **The majority of fungi are:**
   a. Saprophytic
   b. Prokaryotic
   c. Opportunistic
   d. None of these

2. **Dermatophytosis is also called:**
   a. Blastomycosis
   b. Ringworm
   c. Rhabdomycosis
   d. Aflatoxicosis

3. **Dermatophytosis is restricted to:**
   a. Living cornified layers of skin and appendages
   b. Living cornified layers of skin only
   c. Non-living cornified layers of skin and appendages
   d. Non-living cornified layers of skin only

4. **Dermatophytes are classified into how many genera?**
   a. 1
   b. 2
   c. 3
   d. 4

5. **Classical skin lesions of dermatophytes are:**
   a. Peripheral
   b. Central expansion
   c. Peripheral healing and central expansion, producing ring appearance
   d. Peripheral expansion and central healing, producing ring appearance

6. **Dermatophytosis in cattle is caused by:**

   a. *Trichophyton verrucosum*

   b. *Dermatophyton verrucosum*

   c. *Trichophyton canis*

   d. *Microsporum verrucosum*

7. **Lesions of dermatophytosis are:**

   a. Thin, yellowish-brown and asbestos like

   b. Thick, yellowish-brown and asbestos like

   c. Whitish

   d. Pale in colour

8. **Ringworm in equines is caused by:**

   a. *T. verrucosum*

   b. *T. mentagrophytes*

   c. *T. ajello*

   d. *T. equinum*

9. ***T. equinum* is unique because:**

   a. It does not grow in SDA

   b. It does not grow in moist conditions

   c. It does not grow in any other animals

   d. It requires nicotinic acid for its absolute growth

10. **Ringworm of horses is also called:**

    a. Favus

    b. Sporotrichosis

    c. Dermatophytosis

    d. Aspergillosis

11. **The most common dermatophyte in pigs is:**

    a. *M. nanum*

    b. *M. canis*

c. *T. rubrum*

d. *T. verrucosum*

12. **Dermatophytosis is diagnosed using which technique?**

   a. Fungal culture

   b. Wood's lamp test

   c. Gross lesions

   d. Lab tests

13. **Dermatophytes are mostly seen in:**

   a. Apex of hair

   b. Base of hair shaft

   c. Follicular debris

   d. b and c

14. **Decontamination of soil endemic to fungal diseases can be achieved with:**

   a. Phenols

   b. H_2O_2

   c. 3% Formalin

   d. All of these

15. **Mycetoma is a chronic clinical syndrome involving:**

   a. Cutaneous and subcutaneous tissues

   b. Fascia

   c. Bones

   d. All of these

16. **Definitive culture of mycetoma is obtained through:**

   a. FNAC

   b. Blood smear

   c. Culture

   d. Deep biopsy

17. **Rhinosporidiosis is:**

    a. An acute granulomatous disease

    b. A chronic granulomatous disease

    c. An acute disease

    d. A chronic disease

18. **Rhinosporidiosis is caused by:**

    a. *Psuedoallechria*

    b. *Curvularia*

    c. *Maduralla*

    d. *R. seeberi*

19. **Rhinosporidiosis is characterized by:**

    a. Formation of large polyps

    b. Tumours

    c. Papillomas/warts

    d. All of these

20. **Rhinosporidium commonly affects:**

    a. Nose

    b. Teeth

    c. Tongue

    d. Lips

21. **Rhinosporidium's natural habitat is:**

    a. Fresh water

    b. Stagnated water

    c. Polluted water

    d. Mineral water

22. Which is the most frequently affected species for rhino-sporidiosis?

a. Cattle

b. Camels

c. Buffalo

d. Pigs

23. The primary lesion caused by rhinosporidium is what colour?

a. Pink

b. Blue

c. Yellow

d. White

24. What size is a polyp formed by rhinosporidium?

a. 1 cm dia.

b. 1.5 cm dia.

c. 2 cm dia.

d. 3 cm dia.

25. What is the appearance of a growth caused by rhinosporidium?

a. Kiwi-fruit like

b. Turnip-like

c. Drum-like

d. Cauliflower-like

26. Fungal structures of rhinosporidium can be diagnosed by:

a. H&E stain

b. Alcian blue

c. PAS

d. All of these

27. Sporotrichosis is a:

a. Systemic infection

b. Chronic infection

c. Acute infection

d. All of these

28. **Sporotrichosis is caused by**

a. *Sporothrix schenckii*

b. *Sporothrix canis*

c. *Sporothrix bovis*

d. None of these

29. **Sporothrix is a:**

a. Alga

b. Yeast

c. Dimorphic fungus

d. None of these

30. **Sporothrix mostly affects:**

a. Cattle

b. Buffalo

c. Horses

d. Pigs

31. **Sporotrichosis exists in how many forms?**

a. 1

b. 2

c. 3

d. It does not exist

32. **The subcutaneous form of sporotrichosis involves:**

a. Hepatic system

b. The lymphatic system

c. a and b

d. None of these

33. **Nodules of sporotrichosis appears as:**
    a. Purulent centre surrounded by wide band of epithelioid granulation tissue containing giant cells and lymphocytes
    b. Purulent centre surrounded by narrow band of epithelioid granulation tissue containing giant cells and lymphocytes
    c. a and b
    d. None of these

34. **The most specific test for diagnosing sporotrichosis is:**
    a. Latex slide agglutination test
    b. PCR
    c. ELISA
    d. Latex slide agglutination test with immunodiffusion test

35. **Iodide is tried before amphotericin B for treatment of sporotrichosis because of:**
    a. Toxicity
    b. Drug resistance
    c. Drug interactions
    d. a and b

36. **The first described fungus in animals was:**
    a. Dermatophytosis
    b. Sporotrichosis
    c. Aspergillosis
    d. Rhinosporidiosis

37. **Aspergillosis was first described in:**
    a. Ducks
    b. Poultry
    c. Cattle
    d. Pigs

38.   **Aspergillosis is a disease of the:**

   a. Head

   b. Lungs

   c. Liver

   d. Spleen

39.   **Aspergillosis is more common in:**

   a. Layers

   b. Broilers

   c. Breeder hens

   d. Brooding chicks

40.   **Aspergillosis causes:**

   a. High morbidity

   b. High mortality

   c. a and b

   d. None of these

41.   **Most infections of aspergillus are caused by:**

   a. *A. fumigatus*

   b. *A. flavus*

   c. *A. niger*

   d. *A. terreus*

42.   **Avian aspergillosis is also called:**

   a. Brooder pneumonia

   b. Mycotic pneumonia

   c. Both

   d. None of these

43.   **Aspergillus grows within:**

   a. 0 days

   b. 1 day

c. 2 to 3 days

d. 7 days

44. **The primary source of avian aspergillosis is:**

a. Contaminated poultry litter

b. Contaminated water

c. a and b

d. None of these

45. **Aspergillosis affects birds in which age group?**

a. Young

b. Old

c. a and b

d. All age groups

46. **Common clinical signs of aspergillosis are:**

a. Increased respiration

b. Dyspnoea

c. Gasping

d. All of these

47. **In the acute form of aspergillosis we can observe:**

a. White miliary nodules

b. Yellowish-white miliary nodules

c. Pink miliary nodules

d. None of these

48. **Nodules are not formed in which form of aspergillosis?**

a. Acute form

b. Chronic form

c. Peracute pulmonary form

d. Subacute form

49. **Confirmatory diagnosis of aspergillosis is by:**

   a. Presence of mycelial elements

   b. Positive culture

   c. Nodules formation

   d. a and b

50. ***A. fumigatus* can grow up to which temperature?**

   a. 25 °C

   b. 37 °C

   c. 45 °C

   d. Any temperature

51. **Mycotic abortions occur from:**

   a. 1–2 months

   b. 2–4 months

   c. 4–8 months

   d. The 9th month

52. **The most severe changes in cotyledons lead to:**

   a. Necrotizing placentitis

   b. Placentitis

   c. Putrefaction

   d. None of these

53. **PM examination of cattle dead from systemic aspergillosis shows:**

   a. Cavitated sub pleural nodules

   b. Interlobular emphysema in lungs

   c. a and b

   d. None of these

54. **Equine guttural pouch mycosis is caused by:**

   a. *A. nidulans*

   b. *A. fumigatus*

c. *A. flavus*

d. None of these

55. Huttural pouch mycosis is characterized by:

a. Epistaxis

b. Dysphagia

c. Abnormal respiratory sounds

d. All of these

56. Zygomycosis is also known as:

a. Mucormycosis

b. Phycomycosis

c. a and b

d. None of these

57. Swamp cancer is seen in:

a. Equine

b. Bovine

c. Ovine

d. Caprine

58. Swamp cancer is characterized by:

a. White necrotic itchy lesions

b. Yellow necrotic itchy lesions

c. Necrotic lesions

d. Itchy lesions

59. Which larvae are associated with the swamp cancer?

a. *Conidiobolus coronatus*

b. *Habronema megastoma*

c. a and b

d. None of these

60. **Which of these act as a reservoir for swamp cancer?**

a. *Pythium insidiosum*

b. *Conidiobolus coronatus*

c. *Habronema megastoma*

d. *Basidiobolus haptosporus*

61. **Histoplasmosis is a:**

a. Contagious granulomatous disease

b. Non-contagious granulomatous disease

c. Both

d. None of these

62. **Histoplasma is:**

a. Dimorphic fungus

b. Alga

c. Yeast

d. None of these

63. **Histoplasma is:**

a. Capsulated

b. Motile

c. Non-capsulated

d. Non-motile

64. **Histoplasma produces:**

a. Tuberculated chlamydoconidia

b. Massive chlamydoconidia

c. Chlamydoconidia

d. None of these

65. **Histoplasma infection spreads by what means?**

a. Ingestion

b. Fomites

c. Mechanical

d. Inhalation

66. Histoplasma produces no characteristic symptoms in:

a. Cows

b. Horses

c. Dogs

d. Camels

67. Histoplasmosis is confirmed by:

a. PCR

b. ELISA

c. AGPT

d. Mouse inoculation test

68. Disseminated cases of histoplasmosis can be treated with:

a. Amphotericin-B

b. Ketaconazole

c. Itraconazole

d. Meconazole

69. African farcy is also called:

a. Enzootic lymphangitis

b. Epizootic lymphangitis

c. Pseudo glanders

d. b and c

70. Epizootic lymphangitis is a:

a. Acute contagious disease

b. Chronic contagious disease

c. Acute disease

d. Chronic disease

71. *Histoplasma capsulatum* var. *farciminosum* was first known as:

a. *Histoplasma farciminosum*

b. *Cryptococcus farciminosum*

c. a and b

d. None of these

72. **Epizootic lymphangitis has a high infection rate in:**

a. Males

b. Females

c. a and b

d. None of these

73. **Epizootic lymphangitis can be isolated through:**

a. SDA agar

b. Hartley digest medium

c. and b

d. None of these

74. **Gilchrist's disease is also called:**

a. Actinomycosis

b. Dermatophytosis

c. Blastomycosis

d. None of these

75. **Blastomycosis is:**

a. An alga

b. A yeast

c. Conidia

d. Dimorphic fungus

76. **Blastomycosis at 37 °C is:**

a. Yeast form

b. Fungus

c. Mycelium

d. Alga

77. **Blastomycosis at 25 °C is:**

a. Yeast form

b. Mycelium

c. Fungus

d. Alga

78. **Cutaneous lesions of blastomycosis in horses are most common in:**

a. Abdomen

b. Upper legs

c. Lower legs

d. Pelvis

79. **Posads disease is also called:**

a. Rhabdomycosis

b. Actinomycosis

c. Blastomycosis

d. Coccidioidomycosis

80. ***Coccidioides immitis* grows as:**

a. White fluffy mould

b. A non-budding spherical form

c. a and b

d. None of these

81. **Coccidioidomycosis is a:**

a. Benign disease

b. Malignant disease

c. a and b

d. None of these

82. **Confirmation of coccidioidomycosis is performed using:**
    a. AGPT
    b. CFT
    c. RBPT
    d. ELISA

83. **Thrush is also called:**
    a. Candidiasis
    b. Moniliasis
    c. Bronchomycosis
    d. All of these

84. **Candidiasis is a:**
    a. Benign disease
    b. Malignant disease
    c. Sporadic disease
    d. None of these

85. **Candidiasis is caused by:**
    a. *C. albicans*
    b. *C. krusei*
    c. *C. tropicalis*
    d. *C. viswanathii*

86. **Prolonged use of antibiotics leads to:**
    a. Mammalian candidiasis
    b. Avian candidiasis
    c. Bronchomycosis
    d. Blastomycosis

87. **Lesions of candidiasis are mostly seen in:**
    a. Gizzard
    b. Mouth

c. Crop

d. Duodenum

88. **Post-mortem examination of crop of the birds affected with candidiasis reveals:**

a. Turkish towel

b. Hard

c. Smooth

d. None of these

89. **Effective control of candidiasis is achieved by using:**

a. Copper sulfate @ 1:100 dilution

b. Copper sulfate @ 1:200 dilution

c. Copper sulfate @ 1:500 dilution

d. Copper sulfate @ 1:2000 dilution

90. **Candidiasis is rare in:**

a. Equines

b. Bovines

c. Caprines

d. Ovines

91. **Geotrichum is caused by:**

a. *Geotrichum capsulatum*

b. *G. candidum*

c. a and b

d. None of these

92. **Torulosis is also called:**

a. Cryptococcosis

b. European blastomycosis

c. Busse busches disease

d. All of these

93. **Cryptococcosis frequently affects:**

    a. ANS

    b. CNS

    c. a and b

    d. None of these

94. **Cryptococcosis is caused by:**

    a. *Cryptococcus neoformans*

    b. *C. albicans*

    c. *C. capsulatum*

    d. None of these

95. **Adiaspiromycosis is also called:**

    a. Haplomycosis

    b. Adiasporosis

    c. a and b

    d. None of these

96. **The primary cause of mycotic abortion is:**

    a. *Aspergillus fumigatus*

    b. *Candida albicans*

    c. *Coccidioides immitis*

    d. None of these

97. **What is the incidence of mycotic abortion?**

    a. 1%

    b. 3%

    c. 8%

    d. 16%

98. **If the tissue sample of mycotic abortion has to be examined, it must be fixed in:**

    a. 10% Formalin

    b. 10% Phenol

   c. 10% Lyzol

   d. None of these

99. Fungal metabolites are also called:

   a. Ochratoxins

   b. Mycotoxins

   c. Flavotoxins

   d. None of these

100. The Greek word *mykes* means:

   a. Poison

   b. Metabolite

   c. Fungus

   d. All of these

101. The Latin word *toxicum* means:

   a. Poison

   b. Metabolite

   c. Fungus

   d. All of these

102. Mycotoxins are:

   a. Not infectious

   b. Not contagious

   c. a and b

   d. One of these

103. Mycotoxins:

   a. Have low molecular weight

   b. Are non-antigenic

   c. Are not easily destroyed

   d. All of these

104. **Tremorgenic mycotoxicosis contains which mycotoxin?**

   a. Tremorgins

   b. Tremortin

   c. a and b

   d. None of these

105. **Cyclopiazonic acid toxicosis is caused by:**

   a. *A. flavus*

   b. *P. griseofulvin*

   c. *A. coenophialum*

   d. None of these

106. **Cyclopiazonic acid toxicosis causes:**

   a. Liver granulomas

   b. Enteritis

   c. Lymphoid depletion in the spleen

   d. All of these

107. **Lupinosis contains the mycotoxin:**

   a. Phomopsins A

   b. Phomopsins B

   c. a and b

   d. None of these

108. **Fescue toxicity is caused by:**

   a. *A. flavus*

   b. *A. fumigatus*

   c. *Acremonium coenophialum*

   d. *Pithomyces cheratum*

109. **Facial eczema contains which mycotoxin?**

   a. Phomopsins

   b. Tremorgins

    c. Sporodesmin

    d. None of these

110. Toxic hepatitis, cirrhosis and photosensitization are lesions found in:

    a. Facial eczema

    b. Fescue toxicity

    c. Lupinosis

    d. None of these

111. Aflatoxins are:

    a. Nephrotoxic

    b. Hepatotoxic

    c. Ototoxic

    d. Urotoxic

112. The most potent teratogenic and carcinogenic toxin is:

    a. Ochratoxin

    b. Ergotism

    c. Aflatoxin

    d. Tremorgins

113. Aflatoxicosis is caused by:

    a. *A. parasiticus*

    b. *Penicillium puberculum*

    c. *A. nominus*

    d. *A. flavus*

114. Which species is most susceptible to aflatoxicosis?

    a. Poultry

    b. Ducks

    c. Dogs

    d. Cattle

115. **Aflatoxins are:**

    a. Bifurocoumarins

    b. Coumarins

    c. Furocoumarins

    d. Trifurocoumarins

116. **What is the colour fluorescence of aflatoxin B?**

    a. Red

    b. Brown

    c. Blue

    d. Green

117. **Aflatoxin G is:**

    a. Red

    b. Brown

    c. Blue

    d. Green

118. **Which is the correct decreasing order of aflatoxin toxic potency?**

    a. G2, B2, G1, B1

    b. B1, B2, G1, G2

    c. B1, G1, B2, G2

    d. B2, G2, B1, G1

119. **Aflatoxins excreted in milk are referred to as:**

    a. M1, M2

    b. G1, G2

    c. B1, B2

    d. All of these

120. **At which age are calves susceptible to aflatoxicosis?**

    a. 1 month

    b. 3–6 months

c. 1 year

d. 2 years

121. **Aflatoxins lead to the development of:**

   a. Tumours

   b. Abscesses

   c. Haematomas

   d. Cysts

122. **Aflatoxins depress which Ig levels?**

   a. IgA and IgG

   b. IgG and IgM

   c. IgA

   d. IgG

123. **Ochratoxins are produced by:**

   a. *Aspergillus* spp.

   b. *Aspergillus* and *penicillium notatum*

   c. *Penicillium notatum*

   d. All of these

124. **Which ochratoxin is the most toxic?**

   a. A

   b. B

   c. C

   d. D

125. **Which fluorescence is produced by all ochratoxins?**

   a. Bright blue

   b. Green

   c. Blue-green

   d. Bright blue-green

126. **Ochratoxins are:**

    a. Ototoxic

    b. Nephrotoxic

    c. Hepatotoxic

    d. None of these

127. **Which species is most susceptible to ochratoxins?**

    a. Ducks

    b. Geese

    c. Poultry

    d. All birds

128. **Which is a highly potent renal toxin?**

    a. Ochratoxin A

    b. Ochratoxin B

    c. Ochratoxin C

    d. Ochratoxin D

129. **What are the sensitive indicators of ochratoxicosis?**

    a. Serum total protein

    b. Albumin

    c. Serum total protein and albumin

    d. None of these

130. **The largest group of mycotoxins is the:**

    a. Aflatoxins

    b. Trichothecenes

    c. Ergots

    d. Ochratoxins

131. **Stachybotryotoxicosis is caused by:**

    a. *Stachybotrys atra*

    b. Mycothecin

c. a and b

d. None of these

132. Stachybotryotoxicosis in animals causes:

a. Oesophagitis

b. Stomatitis

c. Pharyngitis

d. Choke

133. Stachybotryotoxicosis causes enlargement of which lymph nodes?

a. Mandibular

b. Popliteal

c. Supramammary

d. Submaxillary

134. Myrothecitoxicosis is caused by:

a. *Stachybotrys atra*

b. *Myrothecium roridum*

c. a and b

d. None of these

135. The oldest known mycotoxins are the:

a. Aflatoxins

b. Ochratoxins

c. Ergots

d. None of these

136. Ergotism is caused by:

a. *A. flavus*

b. *A. fumigatus*

c. *Stachybotrys atra*

d. *Claviceps purpurea*

137. **Ergot alkaloids have which property?**

    a. Vasoconstrictor

    b. Vasodilator

    c. Renoconstrictor

    d. Renodilator

138. **Zearaleone toxicity is produced by:**

    a. *A. flavus*

    b. *A. fumigatus*

    c. *Stachybotrys atra*

    d. *Fusarium graminerium*

139. **Which mycotoxin has oestrogenic activity?**

    a. Fusarium

    b. Zearaleone

    c. Aflatoxin

    d. Ochratoxin

140. **Facial eczema is produced by:**

    a. *A. flavus*

    b. *A. fumigatus*

    c. *Pithomyces chartarum*

    d. *Claviceps purpurea*

141. **Fescue toxicity is caused by:**

    a. *A. flavus*

    b. *Acremonium coenophialum*

    c. *Stachybotrys atra*

    d. *Claviceps purpurea*

142. **Equine leukoencephalomalacia is also called:**

    a. Mouldy corn poisoning

    b. Mycotoxin

c. Flavotoxin

d. None of these

143. **Equine leukoencephalomalacia is caused by:**

a. *Fusarium moniliforme*

b. *Acremonium coenophialum*

c. *Stachybotrys atra*

d. *Claviceps purpurea*

144. **Equine leukoencephalomalacia lesions demonstrate:**

a. Coagulative necrosis

b. Necrosis

c. Liquefactive necrosis

d. None of these

145. **Which substance induces the resolution of granulomatous lesions?**

a. Sulphides

b. Chlorides

c. Nitrites

d. Iodides

146. **Which antifungal drug has very broad-spectrum activity**

a. Ketaconazole

b. Itraconazole

c. Meconazole

d. All of these

147. **The dose rate for ketaconazole is:**

a. 5 mg/kg BWT

b. 10 mg/kg BWT

c. 20 mg/kg BWT

d. 30 mg/kg BWT

148. **The dose rate for clotrimazole is:**

   a. 5–10 mg/kg BWT

   b. 10–20 mg/kg BWT

   c. 40–50 mg/kg BWT

   d. 100 mg/kg BWT

149. **The drug of choice for ringworm in small animals is:**

   a. Ketaconazole

   b. Itraconazole

   c. Meconazole

   d. Griseofulvin

150. **The dose rate for griseofulvin is:**

   a. 5 mg/kg BWT

   b. 10 mg/kg BWT

   c. 20 mg/kg BWT

   d. 30 mg/kg BWT

151. **Which antibiotic affects membranes?**

   a. Amphotericin B

   b. Nystatin

   c. Polyenes

   d. All of these

152. **Nystatin is effective in treating which infections?**

   a. Topical yeast infections

   b. Systemic yeast infections

   c. Topical mould infections

   d. Systemic mould infections

153. **The dose rate for nystatin in dogs is:**

   a. 0.5 mg/kg BWT

   b. 0.15 mg/kg BWT

c. 0. 20 mg/kg BWT

d. 0.30 mg/kgBWT

154. Which is an example of a fluorinated pyramidine?

a. Flucytosine

b. Itraconazole

c. Meconazole

d. Griseofulvin

155. The dose rate for flucytosine is:

a. 50 mg/kg BWT

b. 100 mg/kg BWT

c. 150 mg/kg BWT

d. 300 mg/kg BWT

156. Fungi are:

a. Eukaryotic

b. Prokaryotic

c. a and b

d. None of these

157. Fungi are:

a. Motile

b. Non-motile

c. Movable

d. Immovable

158. Fungi reproduce:

a. Sexually

b. Asexually

c. Sexually and asexually

d. None of these

159. **The vegetative structure of a fungus is called the:**

   a. Thallus

   b. Hallus

   c. Callus

   d. All of these

160. **Fungi are usually:**

   a. Aerobic

   b. Anaerobic

   c. Obligate anaerobes

   d. Facultative anaerobes

161. **Obligate or strict anaerobic fungi are found in the:**

   a. Rumen

   b. Reticulum

   c. Omasum

   d. Abomasum

162. **The optimum temperature for saprophytic fungi is:**

   a. 10–30 °C

   b. 22–30 °C

   c. 39–45 °C

   d. 60 °C

163. **The optimum temperature of parasitic fungi is:**

   a. 10–30 °C

   b. 22–30 °C

   c. 39–45 °C

   d. 30–37 °C

164. **Which pH is preferred by most fungi?**

   a. Alkaline

   b. Neutral

c. Acidic

d. None of these

165. The optimum pH range for growth of fungi is:

a. 0

b. 1–2

c. 2–3

d. 3.8–5.6

**166. The budding type of multiplication produces......................
consistency ?**

a. Pasty

b. Mucoid

c. Pasty to mucoid

d. None of these

167. Monomorphic yeasts include:

a. *Candida albicans*

b. *Cryptococcus neoformans*

c. *Geotrichum candidurn*

d. All of these

168. Hyphae may become:

a. Septate

b. Branched

c. a and b

d. None of these

169. Hyphae develop into a mat of filamentous growth known as:

a. Mycelium

b. Septate

c. Budding

d. None of these

170. **Monomorphic moulds include:**

   a. Microsporum

   b. Trichophyton

   c. Aspergillus

   d. all of these

171. **Dimorphic fungi include:**

   a. *Histoplasma capsulatum*

   b. *Blastomyces dermatitidis*

   c. *Sporothrix schenckii*

   d. All of these

172. **The presence of cross walls in a hyphal filament is known as:**

   a. Septate

   b. Aseptate

   c. Pseudo-hyphae

   d. None of these

173. **The absence of cross walls in a hyphal filament is known as:**

   a. Septate

   b. Aseptate

   c. Pseudo-hyphae

   d. None of these

174. **A chain of elongated budding cells that have failed to detach is known as:**

   a. Septate

   b. Aseptate

   c. Pseudo-hyphae

   d. None of these

175. **A multicellular conidium is known as a:**

   a. Macroconidium

   b. Microconidium

    c. Chlamydospore

    d. Arthrospore

176. A small, single-celled conidium is known as a:

    a. Macroconidium

    b. Microconidium

    c. Chlamydospore

    d. Arthrospore

177. Thick-walled, resistant spores formed by the direct differentiation of the mycelium are called:

    a. Macroconidiums

    b. Microconidiums

    c. Chlamydospores

    d. Arthrospores

178. Asexual spores formed by the disarticulation of mycelium are called:

    a. Macroconidiums

    b. Microconidiums

    c. Chlamydospores

    d. Arthrospores

179. An example of a chlamydospore is:

    a. *Candida albicans*

    b. *Geotrichum candidum*

    c. *Saccharomyces* spp.

    d. None of these

180. An example of an arthrospore is:

    a. *Candida albicans*

    b. *Geotrichum candidum*

    c. *Saccharomyces* spp.

    d. None of these

181. **An example of a blastospore is:**

    a. *Candida albicans*

    b. *Geotrichum candidum*

    c. *Saccharomyces* spp.

    d. None of these

182. **An asexual spore produced by closed, often spherical structures is called a:**

    a. Macroconidium

    b. Microconidium

    c. Chlamydospore

    d. Sporangiospore

183. **An example of a sporangiospore is:**

    a. *Rhizopus*

    b. *Candida albicans*

    c. *Geotrichum candidum*

    d. *Saccharomyces* spp.

184. **The dome-shaped upper portion of a sporangiophore is called the:**

    a. Columella

    b. Macroconidium

    c. Microconidium

    d. Chlamydospore

185. **A sexual spore characteristic of the true yeasts and the class Ascomycetes is:**

    a. Ascospore

    b. Basidiospore

    c. Zygospore

    d. Gametangium

186. **Ascospores are produced in a sac-like structure called a:**

a. Ascus

b. Basidium

c. Gametangium

d. None of these

187. **An example of an ascospore is:**

a. *Candida albicans*

b. *Geotrichum candidum*

c. *Saccharomyces* spp.

d. None of these

188. **A sexual spore characteristic of the class Basidiomycetes is:**

a. Ascospore

b. Basidiospore

c. Zygospore

d. Gametangium

189. **What is the name for a basidiospore produced on a specialized club-like structure?**

a. Ascus

b. Basidium

c. Gametangium

d. None of these

190. **What is the name for a thick-walled sexual spore produced through fusion of two similar gametangia?**

a. Ascospore

b. Basidiospore

c. Zygospore

d. Gametangium

191. **What is the name for a structure in which gametes are produced?**

    a. Ascospore

    b. Basidiospore

    c. Zygospore

    d. Gametangium

192. **What is the name for a sexual cell, especially a cell formed in a gametangium?**

    a. Ascospore

    b. Basidiospore

    c. Zygospore

    d. Gamete

193. **What is the name for a stalk-like branch of the mycelium on which conidia develop either singly or in multiples?**

    a. Conidiophore

    b. Sporangiophore

    c. a and b

    d. None of these

194. **A specialised hypha-bearing sporangium is known as a:**

    a. Conidiophore

    b. Sporangiophore

    c. a and b

    d. None of these

195. **An example of a 'perfect' fungus is:**

    a. *Candida albicans*

    b. *Geotrichum candidum*

    c. *Saccharomyces* spp.

    d. None of these

196. **'Imperfect' fungi belong to the class:**

   a. Deuteromycetes

   b. Actinomycetes

   c. Basidiomycetes

   d. None of these

197. **The most primitive class of fungi are the:**

   a. Phycomycetes

   b. Ascomycetes

   c. Basidiomycetes

   d. Deuteromycetes

198. **Which is an example of superficial mycosis?**

   a. *Trichosporon cutaneum*

   b. *Candida albicans*

   c. *Rhinosporidium seebri*

   d. Cryptococcosis

199. **Which is an example of cutaneous mycosis?**

   a. *Trichosporon cutaneum*

   b. *Candida albicans*

   c. *Rhinosporidium seebri*

   d. Cryptococcosis

200. **Which is an example of subcutaneous mycosis?**

   a. *Trichosporon cutaneum*

   b. *Candida albicans*

   c. *Rhinosporidium seebri*

   d. Cryptococcosis

201. **Which is an example of systemic mycosis?**

   a. *Trichosporon cutaneum*

   b. *Candida albicans*

   c. *Rhinosporidium seebri*

   d. Cryptococcosis

202. **Most fungal diseases are not contagious or zoonotic except:**

   a. Dermatophytosis

   b. Aspergillosis

   c. Rhinosporidiosis

   d. All of these

203. ***Trichophyton mentagrophytes* affects:**

   a. All domestic animals

   b. Cattle and sheep

   c. Fowl

   d. Horses

204. ***Trichophyton verrucosum* affects:**

   a. All domestic animals

   b. Cattle and sheep

   c. Fowl

   d. Horses

205. ***Trichophyton gallinae* affects:**

   a. All domestic animals

   b. Cattle and sheep

   c. Fowl

   d. Horses

206. ***Trichophyton equinum* affects:**

   a. All domestic animals

   b. Cattle and sheep

   c. Fowl

   d. Horses

207. *Microsporum canis* mainly affects:

a. Dogs and cats

b. Primates

c. Horses

d. All of these

208. *Microsporum nanum* affects:

a. All domestic animals

b. Cattle and sheep

c. Fowl

d. Swine and humans

209. An example of a geophilic pathogen is:

a. *Microsporum gypseum*

b. *Trichophyton mentagrophytes*

c. *Microsporum canis*

d. *Microsporum nanum*

210. The most common media for propagating dermatophytes is:

a. Dermatophyte test medium (DTM) or Sabouraud's dextrose agar

b. 2% agar containing 1% peptone

c. 4% glucose

d. All of these

211. Dermatophytes are:

a. Bacteriostatic

b. Bacteriocidal

c. Mildly bacteriostatic

d. Mildly bacteriocidal

212. *Microsporum* is visible under:

a. Wood's lamp test

b. PCR

c. ELISA

d. All of these

213. **Which proteolytic enzyme determines virulence, particularly in severe inflammatory disease of dermatophytes?**

a. Elastase

b. Collagenase

c. Keratinase

d. all of these

214. **A clearly recognized virulence factor for dermatophytes is:**

a. Keratinase

b. Lipase

c. Peptidase

d. None of these

215. **Dermatophytes are:**

a. Low species-specific

b. Highly species-specific

c. Moderately species-specific

d. None of these

216. **Tinea barabe affects:**

a. Beard

b. Scalp

c. Body

d. Groin

217. **Tinea capitis affects:**

a. Beard

b. Scalp

c. Body

d. Groin

218. **Tinea corporis affects:**

a. Beard

b. Scalp

c. Body

d. Groin

219. **Tinea cruris affects:**

a. Beard

b. Scalp

c. Body

d. Groin

220. **Tinea favosa affects:**

a. Scalp

b. Hands

c. Feet

d. Nails

221. **Tinea imbricata and Tinea manum affect:**

a. Scalp

b. Hands

c. Feet

d. Nails

222. **Tinea pedis affects:**

a. Scalp

b. Hands

c. Feet

d. Nails

223. **Tinea unguium affects:**

a. Scalp

b. Hands

c. Feet

d. Nails

224. Crop mycosis or Avian moniliasis affects:

a. Chickens

b. Turkeys

c. Poultry

d. All of these

225. Stomach ulcers and cutaneous candidiasis appear in:

a. Chickens

b. Swine

c. Poultry

d. All of these

226. Mycotic stomatitis as well as enteritis in candidiasis appear in:

a. Puppies and kittens

b. Calves

c. Foals

d. All of these

227. Genital tract infection caused by candidiasis is seen in

a. Mares

b. Bitches

c. a and b

d. None of these

228. Chlamydospores on cornmeal agar is seen in:

a. *C. albicans*

b. *C. tropicalis*

c. *C. pseudotropicalis*

d. *C. parapsilosis*

229. **Subcutaneous and nasal granulomas, meningitis and blindness are seen in:**

    a. Dogs and cats

    b. Horses

    c. Cattle

    d. Humans

230. **Nasal granuloma is seen in:**

    a. Dogs and cats

    b. Horses

    c. Cattle

    d. Humans

231. **Cryptococcal mastitis is seen in:**

    a. Dogs and cats

    b. Horses

    c. Cattle

    d. Humans

232. **Cryptococcal meningitis is seen in:**

    a. Dogs and cats

    b. Horses

    c. Cattle

    d. Humans

233. **How is histoplasma stained?**

    a. Using gomori methanamine

    b. Using periodic acid-schiff stains

    c. a and b

    d. None of these

234. **Acute aspergillosis appears in:**

    a. Avians

    b. Bovines

  c. Ovines

  d. Equines

235. **Abortion, pneumonia and mastitis caused by aspergillosis is seen in**

  a. Avians

  b. Bovines

  c. Ovines

  d. Equines

236. **Pneumonia and abortion caused by aspergillosis is seen in**

  a. Avians

  b. Bovines

  c. Ovines

  d. Equines

237. **Abortion and diarrhoea caused by aspergillosis is seen in**

  a. Avians

  b. Bovines

  c. Ovines

  d. Equines

238. **Ear and nasal infections by *Aspergillus* are seen in :**

  a. Avians

  b. Bovines

  c. Ovines

  d. Equines

239. **Fatal pulmonary aspergillosis by *Aspergillus* is seen in**

  a. Avians

  b. Bovines

  c. Canines

  d. Felines

240. **A velvety or powdery, at first white, then turning to dark bluish-green morphology is seen in:**

a. *A. fumigatus*

b. *A. niger*

c. *A. flavus*

d. None of these

241. **A woolly, at first white to yellow and then turning dark brown to black morphology is seen in:**

a. *A. fumigatus*

b. *A. niger*

c. *A. flavus*

d. None of these

242. **A velvety, yellow to green or brown morphology is seen in:**

a. *A. fumigatus*

b. *A. niger*

c. *A. flavus*

d. None of these

243. **Aflatoxins can be revealed by:**

a. Thin layer chromatography

b. Thick layer chromatography

c. a and b

d. None of these

244. **Aflatoxins mostly affect the:**

a. Vascular system

b. Digestive system

c. Mucus membrane

d. a and b

245. **Trichothecane (t-2) toxin mostly affects:**

a. The vascular system

b. The digestive system

c. The mucus membranes

d. The urinary system

246. **Ochratoxin mostly affects:**

a. The vascular system

b. The digestive system

c. The mucus membranes

d. The urinary system

247. **Zearalenone mostly affects:**

a. The vascular system

b. The digestive system

c. The mucus membranes

d. The urinary system

248. **Sporidesmin mostly affects:**

a. The vascular system

b. The digestive system

c. The mucus membranes

d. The urinary system

249. **Aflatoxins are:**

a. Carcinogenic

b. Teratogenic

c. Mutagenic

d. All of these

250. **Acute toxicity of aflatoxin causes:**

a. Hepatic injury

b. Ataxia

c. Convulsions

d. All of these

Answers

1.	a	32.	b	63.	c	94.	a
2.	b	33.	a	64.	a	95.	c
3.	c	34.	d	65.	d	96.	a
4.	c	35.	d	66.	c	97.	d
5.	d	36.	c	67.	d	98.	a
6.	a	37.	a	68.	a	99.	b
7.	b	38.	b	69.	b	100.	c
8.	c	39.	d	70.	b	101.	a
9.	d	40.	c	71.	c	102.	c
10.	a	41.	a	72.	a	103.	d
11.	a	42.	a	73.	b	104.	c
12.	b	43.	c	74.	c	105.	b
13.	d	44.	a	75.	d	106.	d
14.	c	45.	d	76.	a	107.	c
15.	d	46.	d	77.	b	108.	c
16.	d	47.	b	78.	c	109.	c
17.	b	48.	c	79.	d	110.	a
18.	d	49.	d	80.	c	111.	b
19.	d	50.	c	81.	a	112.	c
20.	a	51.	c	82.	b	113.	d
21.	b	52.	a	83.	d	114.	b
22.	c	53.	c	84.	c	115.	a
23.	d	54.	b	85.	a	116.	c
24.	d	55.	d	86.	b	117.	d
25.	d	56.	c	87.	c	118.	c
26.	d	57.	a	88.	a	119.	a
27.	b	58.	b	89.	d	120.	b
28.	a	59.	c	90.	a	121.	c
29.	c	60.	d	91.	b	122.	a
30.	c	61.	b	92.	d	123.	b
31.	b	62.	a	93.	b	124.	a

(Continued)

125.	d	157.	b	189.	b	221.	b
126.	b	158.	c	190.	c	222.	c
127.	c	159.	a	191.	d	223.	d
128.	a	160.	a	192.	d	224.	d
129.	c	161.	a	193.	a	225.	b
130.	b	162.	b	194.	b	226.	d
131.	a	163.	d	195.	c	227.	c
132.	b	164.	c	196.	a	228.	a
133.	d	165.	d	197.	a	229.	a
134.	b	166.	c	198.	a	230.	b
135.	c	167.	d	199.	b	231.	c
136.	d	168.	c	200.	c	232.	d
137.	a	169.	a	201.	d	233.	c
138.	d	170.	d	202.	a	234.	a
139.	b	171.	d	203.	a	235.	b
140.	c	172.	a	204.	b	236.	c
141.	b	173.	b	205.	c	237.	d
142.	a	174.	c	206.	d	238.	c
143.	b	175.	a	207.	d	239.	d
144.	c	176.	b	208.	d	240.	a
145.	d	177.	c	209.	a	241.	b
146.	a	178.	d	210.	d	242.	c
147.	b	179.	a	211.	a	243.	a
148.	c	180.	b	212.	a	244.	a
149.	d	181.	c	213.	d	245.	c
150.	b	182.	d	214.	a	246.	d
151.	d	183.	a	215.	b	247.	d
152.	a	184.	a	216.	a	248.	c
153.	b	185.	a	217.	b	249.	d
154.	a	186.	a	218.	c	250.	d
155.	b	187.	c	219.	d		
156.	a	188.	b	220.	a		

5 Mycoplasma Diseases

J.B. Kathiriya

Introduction

Mycoplasma spp. is a bacteria that can infect various body parts. The type of mycoplasma bacteria decides the area of the body affected. However, all infections have one thing in common: contrary to other bacteria, mycoplasma do not have cell walls and in comparison to other bacteria are very small. Mycoplasmas have a global distribution causing serious diseases in cattle worldwide including mastitis, arthritis, pneumonia, otitis media and reproductive disorders. *Mycoplasma* species are typically highly contagious, are capable of causing severe disease and are difficult infections to resolve, requiring rapid and accurate diagnosis to prevent and control outbreaks. This chapter's questions focus on the development and use of different diagnostic methods to identify mycoplasmas relevant to cattle, with a particular focus on *Mycoplasma bovis*. Mycoplasmas are the smallest of free-living organisms and are intermediate between viruses and bacteria. Many species thrive as parasites in animal (including human) hosts. Traditionally, the identification and diagnosis of *Mycoplasma* has been performed via microbial culture. More recently, the use of polymerase chain reaction to detect *Mycoplasma* species from various bovine samples has increased. Polymerase chain reaction has a higher efficiency, specificity and sensitivity for laboratory diagnosis when compared with conventional culture-based methods. Several tools are now available for typing *Mycoplasma* spp. isolates, allowing for genetic characterization in disease outbreak investigations. Serological diagnosis through the use of indirect ELISA allows the detection of anti-mycoplasma antibodies in sera and milk, with their use demonstrated on individual animal samples as well as BTM samples. While each testing method has strengths and limitations, their combined use provides complementary information which, when interpreted in conjunction with clinical signs and herd history, facilitates pathogen detection and characterization of the disease status of cattle populations.

Multiple Choice Questions

1. **Which of the following stains is used for Mycoplasma?**

   a. Fontana

   b. Diene's

   c. Acid fast

   d. Machiavello

2. **Which bacteria require a living medium for growth?**

   a. Mycoplasma and Leptospira

   b. Chlamydia and Rickettsia

   c. Rickettsia and Mycoplasma

   d. None of these

3. **Mycoplasma organisms are pleomorphic in nature due to:**

   a. Absence of cell wall

   b. Absence of rigid cell wall

   c. Small size

   d. Species specific characteristics

4. **A typical of 'fried egg' appearance colony morphology is a diagnostic feature of:**

   a. *Salmonella Pullorum*

   b. *Salmonella Gallinarum*

   c. Avian pathogenic *E. Coli*

   d. *Mycoplasma gallisepticum*

5. **Pink eye is caused by:**

   a. Moraxella

   b. Chlamydia

   c. Mycoplasma

   d. All of these

6. **The drug of choice for atypical pneumonia due to *Mycoplasma pneumoniae* is:**

    a. Doxycycline

    b. Ciprofloxacin

    c. Ceftriaxone

    d. Gentamicin

7. **Which bacteria requires the X and V factor for growth in the medium?**

    a. Haemophilus

    b. Moraxella

    c. Mycoplasma

    d. a and c

8. **Which of the following organisms is sensitive to digitoxin?**

    a. Mycoplasma

    b. Acholeplasma

    c. a and b

    d. None of these

9. **Which bacteria require cholesterol for growth?**

    a. Leptospira

    b. Mycoplasma

    c. Spirochaete

    d. None of these

10. **Mycoplasma in poultry causes:**

    a. Fowl typhoid

    b. Fowl cholera

    c. Fowl plague

    d. CRD

11. **Which factor is able to aggravate postvaccinal reaction?**

   a. *E. coli*

   b. Low relative humidity

   c. *Mycoplasma gallispticum*

   d. All of these

12. **Characteristic features of fowl mycoplasmosis are:**

   a. White fibrinous membrane on the surface of liver

   b. Pericarditis

   c. Perihepatitis

   d. Air sacculitis

13. **Mycoplasmosis is also known as:**

   a. CRD

   b. Air sac disease

   c. a and b

   d. Aftosa

14. **In poultry, what is affected in cases of CRD?**

   a. Upper respiratory tract

   b. Lower respiratory tract

   c. Beak

   d. All of these

15. ***Mycoplasma* spp. was probably first encountered in chicks by:**

   a. Nelsen

   b. Koch

   c. Virchow

   d. Jenner

16. **Which disease of poultry is caused by Mycoplama?**

   a. Chronic respiratory disease

   b. Infectious coryza

c. Chicken infectious anaemia

d. Avian encephalomyelitis

17. **Infectious sinusitis caused by *Mycoplasma* spp. is most commonly seen in:**

a. Chickens

b. Turkeys

c. Dogs

d. Sheep

18. **Rolling disease in mice is caused by:**

a. *Mycoplasma neurolyticum*

b. *Corynebacterium*

c. *Klebsiella pneumoniae*

d. *Campylobacter*

19. **Eaton's agent is a synonym for:**

a. *Corynebacterium*

b. *Klebsiella pneumoniae*

c. *Streptococcus pyogens*

d. *Mycoplasma pneumoniae*

20. **The drug of choice for mycoplasmosis is:**

a. Tylosin

b. Buparvaquone

c. Gentamicin

d. Ceftriaxone

21. **Which medium is used to grow Mycoplasma?**

a. PPLO agar

b. Frey's medium

c. a and b

d. None of these

22. **Which of these is not related to Mycoplasma?**

   a. CCPP

   b. CRD

   c. CBPP

   d. BSE

23. **Mycoplasma is:**

   a. Eukaryotic and unicellular

   b. Prokaryotic and unicellular

   c. Prokaryotic and multicellular

   d. Eukaryotic and multicellular

24. **Which is the smallest organism capable of autonomous growth and reproduction?**

   a. Mycoplasma

   b. Virus

   c. Viroid

   d. None of these

25. **Mycoplasmas can be cultivated *in vitro* on nonliving media as:**

   a. Facultative aerobes

   b. Facultative anaerobes

   c. Obligate aerobes

   d. Microaerophiles

26. **What type of colony is formed by Mycoplasmas on agar plate?**

   a. Colourless

   b. Lawn formation

   c. Coloured

   d. Fried egg

27.   **Mycoplasma is:**

a. Eukaryotic and unicellular

b. Prokaryotic and unicellular

c. Prokaryotic and multicellular

d. Eukaryotic and multicellular

28.   **The 'witch's broom' of legumes is caused by a:**

a. Fungus

b. Bacterium

c. Mycoplasma

d. Virus

29.   **Which species of Mycoplasma causes human sterility?**

a. *T. mycoplasma*

b. *M. fermentans*

c. *M. hominis*

d. All of these

30.   **In Mycoplasma, the elementary cell body performs the function of:**

a. Respiration

b. Reproduction

c. Excretion

d. Metabolism

31.   **What are known as the 'Jokers of the microbiological park'?**

a. Nostoc

b. Mycoplasma

c. Bacteria

d. None of these

32.   **Which are osmotically inactive?**

a. Nostoc

b. Mycoplasma

   c. Bacteria

   d. All of these

33. **Vancomycin and penicillin do not affect Mycoplasma because:**

   a. There is no Golgi body

   b. There are no mitochondria

   c. There is no nucleus

   d. There is no cell wall

34. **Which bacteria is without a cell wall?**

   a. Cyanobacteria

   b. Mycoplasma

   c. Viroid

   d. Virus

35. **'Little leaf of brinjal' is caused by:**

   a. Algae

   b. Fungus

   c. Mycoplasma

   d. Virus

36. **The characteristic feature of eubacteria is:**

   a. Rigid cell wall

   b. Flagellum in motile ones

   c. Chlorophyll a

   d. All of these

37. **Which of the following are common human infections caused by *Mycoplasma* spp.?**

   a. Pneumonia

   b. Food poisoning

   c. Urethritis

   d. a and c

38. **Which of these is not a general characteristic of *Mycoplasma* spp.?**

    a. It can grow on cell-free media containing lipoprotein and sterol

    b. It is pleomorphic and very small in size

    c. It is best identified using a gram staining technique

    d. In media, colonies appear as a fried egg in shape

39. **A 14-year-old boy contracts cough and fever at school where one of his friends from the class had the same symptoms for a few days. At the hospital, laboratory sputum culture and gram staining methods show negative results and chest radiography does not show the infection area properly. Which is the likely pathogen?**

    a. *Mycoplasma hominis*

    b. *Mycoplasma pneumoniae*

    c. *Mycobacterium leprae*

    d. *Ureaplasma urealyticum*

40. **Which of the following statements is true about *Ureaplasma urealyticum*?**

    a. It can be cultivated in a routine culture medium

    b. The transmission of the bacteria is through the respiratory passage

    c. The bacteria can grow easily in media containing urea

    d. It is susceptible to penicillin and amoxicillin

41. **_Mycoplasma_ spp. are resistant to penicillin:**

    a. True

    b. False

42. **A blood sample from a 19-year-old sexually active woman with genital infections is taken and cultured for the isolation of the responsible pathogen. Name the least likely pathogen that might be responsible for the infection?**

    a. *Chlamydia trachomatis*

    b. *Mycoplasma hominis*

c. *Mycoplasma pneumoniae*

d. *Mycoplasma genitalium*

43. **Select the primary pathogen(s) of genital infections:**

a. *Mycoplasma pneumoniae*

b. *Mycoplasma hominis*

c. *Ureaplasma urealyticum*

d. b and c

44. **The routine laboratory diagnostics method is usually not helpful for the isolation and identification of *Mycoplasma pneumoniae*. All of the following are important clinical tests for the diagnosis of the infection in humans except:**

a. ELISA

b. Complement fixation

c. Cold hemagglutinins

d. Electron microscopy

45. **Which of the following pathogens commonly cause community-acquired pneumonia?**

a. *Streptococcus pneumoniae*

b. *Mycoplasma pneumoniae*

c. *Haemophilus influenza*

d. All of these

46. **Which of the following Mollicutes is associated with the infection salpingitis and postpartum fevers?**

a. *Mycoplasma genitalium*

b. *Ureaplasma urealyticum*

c. *Mycoplasma hominis*

d. *Mycoplasma pneumonia*

47. **Which of the following *Mycoplasma* spp. grow rapidly in broth and agar mediums?**

    a. *Ureaplasma urealyticum*

    b. *Mycoplasma genitalium*

    c. *Mycoplasma pneumoniae*

    d. None of these

48. **_Ureaplasma urealyticum_ is found as normal flora in the urinary tract in sexually active men and women. About what percentage of women have it?**

    a. 20–40%

    b. 40–80%

    c. 5–20%

    d. 25–45%

49. **_Mycoplasma pneumoniae_ infections are most prevalent in what age group of people?**

    a. 15–60

    b. 5–45

    c. 5–20

    d. 10–50

50. **Which of the following statements is true regarding the pathogenesis of mycoplasma infections?**

    a. Adherence to the host cells is mediated by the bacterial proteins

    b. The bacteria enter the host cell by releasing exotoxin

    c. They are inhibited by beta-lactam antibiotics

    d. All of these

51. **Which of the following is the drug of choice for _Ureaplasma urealyticum_ infections?**

    a. Penicillin

    b. Tetracyclines

    c. Cephalosporins

    d. Imipenem

52. **Which of the following virulence factors is present in *Myco-plasma pneumoniae*, also known as community-acquired distress syndrome toxin?**

    a. Endotoxin

    b. Capsule

    c. Lipid

    d. Exotoxin

53. ***Mycoplasma pneumoniae* can cause extrapulmonary infections and can infect mucous membranes and cutaneous membranes. Symptoms usually include rashes, soreness and inflammation of these membranes. What is the commonly used term for this type of infection?**

    a. Sporotrichosis

    b. Epiglottitis

    c. Mucositis

    d. Cellulitis

54. **What are the different types of infections commonly associated with *M. genitalium*?**

    a. Nongonococcal urethritis in men and women

    b. Pelvic inflammatory disease in women

    c. Infertility in women

    d. All of these

55. **Due to the lack of cell wall, penicillin is not effective against *M. genitalium*, and the bacteria have shown high resistance to azithromycin and other macrolides. Which drug is used for the treatment of infections associated with *M. genitalium*?**

    a. Moxifloxacin

    b. Ceftriaxone

    c. Acyclovir

    d. Retrovir

56. **Which bacteria are resistant to penicillin because it lacks a cell wall?**

a. Spirochetes

b. Cyanobacteria

c. Mycoplasmas

d. Bdellovibrios

57. **The smallest cells of mycoplasmas are of what diameter?**

a. 1 micrometre

b. 0.3 micrometres

c. 5 micrometres

d. 1 metre

58. **Penicillin causes inhibition of mycoplasmas:**

a. True

b. False

59. **Mycoplasmas can be cultivated *in vitro* on nonliving media as:**

a. Facultative aerobes

b. Obligate aerobes

c. Facultative anaerobes

d. Microaerophiles

60. **Agar plate colonies of Mycoplasma can be observed by means of:**

a. A low-power microscope

b. A high-power microscope

c. Phase contrast microscopy

d. Bright field microscopy

61. **The outermost limiting layer of Mycoplasma is made up of:**

a. Cell wall

b. Cell membrane

c. Mucilaginous sheath

d. Slime layer

62. **Mycoplasmas require which of the following substances for growth?**

a. Nitrogen

b. Carbon

c. Cholesterol

d. Glucose

63. **Which of the following families of bacteria are pathogenic for citrus and other plants?**

a. Mycoplasmataceae

b. Acholeplasmataceae

c. Spiroplamataceae

d. Anaplasmataceae

64. ***Lyticum flagellatum* is an endosymbiont carried by certain strains of:**

a. Bacteria

b. Fungi

c. Viruses

d. Protozoa

65. ***L. flagellatum* performs the function of synthesizing:**

a. Vitamins

b. Hormones

c. Organic acids

d. Folic acid and toxins

66. **Mycoplasmas cannot give rise to walled bacterial forms such as L-phase variants:**

a. True

b. False

67. **Which of the following is not a feature of Mycoplasma?**

    a. Cannot live without oxygen

    b. Spherical to filamentous cells with no cell walls

    c. Fried-egg shaped colonies

    d. Lack a nucleus, endoplasmic reticulum, mitochondria and plastids

68. **Which of the following is a prokaryote?**

    a. Bacteria

    b. Mycoplasma

    c. Blue-green algae

    d. All of these

69. **Which microbial agent does not cause atypical pneumonia?**

    a. *Mycoplasma pneumoniae*

    b. *Legionella pneumophila*

    c. Human coronavirus

    d. *Klebsiellapneumonia*

70. **What is produced by gram-positive bacteria where there is a complete absence of cell wall?**

    a. L-form

    b. Spheroplast

    c. Protoplast

    d. Mycoplasma

71. **Which of the following is acid-fast positive?**

    a. Mycoplasma

    b. Nocardia

    c. Neisseria

    d. Fusobacterium

72. **Which of these contains sterol in the cytoplasmic membrane?**

    a. Spirochetes

    b. Mycoplasma

c. Chlamydia

d. Clostridia

73. **What are also known as PPLO?**

a. Rickettsiae

b. Mycoplasma

c. Mycobacteria

d. Chlamydia

74. **Which one of the following statements is wrong?**

a. Golden algae are also called desmids

b. Eubacteria are also called false bacteria

c. Phycomycetes are also called algal fungi

d. Cyanobacteria are also called blue-green algae

75. **Which of the following is called "Jockers of microbiological park"?**

a. Bacteria

b. Fungi

c. Mycoplasma

d. Nostoc

76. **Satellite growth on a blood agar plate in the presence of *Staph. aureus* is characteristic of:**

a. *Pasteurella*

b. *Haemophillus*

c. *Actinobacillus*

d. *Mycoplasma*

77. **Crop mycosis in poultry is caused by:**

a. Bacteria

b. Mycoplasma

c. Fungi

d. Virus

78. **What is the primary mode of reproduction for Mycoplasma?**

    a. Mitosis

    b. Binary fission

    c. Meiosis

    d. Sexual

79. **What type of cell wall do Mycoplasma species lack?**

    a. Peptidoglycan

    b. Cellulose

    c. Chitin

    d. Lignin

80. **Mycoplasma species are known to cause what types of infections in humans?**

    a. Respiratory

    b. Gastrointestinal

    c. Skin

    d. All of these

81. **Mycoplasma reproduces through:**

    a. Sexual means

    b. Asexual means

    c. Vegetative means

    d. No reproduction

82. **What type of environment is most conducive for the growth of Mycoplasma?**

    a. High humidity and warm temperatures

    b. Low humidity and cold temperatures

    c. Neutral pH

    d. High pH

83. **What is the primary method of treatment for Mycoplasma infections?**

    a. Antibiotics

    b. Vaccines

    c. Herbal remedies

    d. None of these

84. **What are the primary symptoms of a Mycoplasma infection?**

    a. Fever and cough

    b. Diarrhoea and vomiting

    c. Rash and itching

    d. All of the above

85. **How do Mycoplasma species obtain energy?**

    a. Aerobic respiration

    b. Anaerobic respiration

    c. Fermentation

    d. Photosynthesis

86. **What is the primary mode of transmission for Mycoplasma infections?**

    a. Direct contact

    b. Indirect contact

    c. Airborne

    d. All of these

87. **What is the primary mechanism of resistance to antibiotics in Mycoplasma?**

    a. Efflux pumps

    b. Enzymatic degradation

    c. Mutations in target genes

    d. All of these

88.   Mycoplasmas are associated with which of the following?

a. Gram-positive cell walls

b. The kingdom of Archaea

c. Cells with a prokaryotic organization

d. A susceptibility to cell lysis in hypotonic solutions

89.   What is the most common cause of atypical pneumonia?

a. *Chlamydophila pneumoniae*

b. *Coxiella burnetii*

c. *Mycoplasma pneumoniae*

d. Influenza

90.   Mycoplasmas are associated with which of the following? Please select all that apply.

a. Gram-positive cell walls

b. The Kingdom of Archaea

c. Cells with a prokaryotic organization

d. A susceptibility to cell lysis in hypotonic solutions

91.   Pneumococcal pneumonia is caused by:

a. *Chlamydophila pneumoniae*

b. *Coxiella burnetii*

c. *Mycoplasma pneumoniae*

d. *Streptococcus pneumoniae*

92.   Mycoplasmas are also known as:

a. Bacteria

b. Cytolysis

c. Achaea

d. Flagella

93.   Elementary cell bodies in Mycoplasma perform the function of:

a. Metabolism

b. Reproduction

    c. Respiration

    d. Excretion

94. **Kuru disease in humans is caused by:**

    a. Bacteria

    b. Viroides

    c. Prions

    d. Mycoplasma

95. **L-lysine is produced from:**

    a. *Coryne bacterium glutamicum*

    b. *Coryne bacterium* spp.

    c. *Mycobacterium* spp.

    d. None of these

96. **Which viruses are known to infect Mycoplasmas?**

    a. Bacteriophages

    b. Mycoplasma phages

    c. Virions

    d. Tiny strain

97. **Which are the drugs of choice for treatment of Mycoplasma infections?**

    a. Tetracyclines

    b. Erythromycin

    c. a and b

    d. Penicillins

98. **Which of the following diseases is not caused by Mycoplasma?**

    a. Pneumonia in human beings

    b. Little leaf of Brinjal

    c. Dwarf disease of Mulberry

    d. Citrus canker

99. **Blebs can be noted in:**

    a. *Mycoplasma galisepticum*

    b. *Spirogyra*

    c. *Pseudomonas cola*

    d. None of these

100. **Accridine dyes are more effective against:**

    a. Gram-positive

    b. Gram-negative

    c. Mycoplasmas

    d. Rickttsiae

101. **Mycoplasmas differ from Chalamydiae in that they:**

    a. Cause urinary tract infections

    b. Lack a true bacterial cell wall

    c. Are susceptible to penicillin

    d. All of these

102. **Who recorded pleuropneumonia in cattle?**

    a. Pasteur

    b. Twort

    c. Knoll and Ruska

    d. Nocard and Roux

103. **Which of the following organisms is most commonly associated with AIDS pneumonia?**

    a. Klebsiella

    b. *Str. pneumonia*

    c. Mycoplasma

    d. *Mycobacterium tuberculosis*

104. **Which of the species of Mycoplasma causes human sterility?**

    a. *M. hominis*

    b. *M. fermentans*

c. *T. mycoplasma*

d. All the three

105. Mycoplasma can live successfully in phloem due to being

a. Osmotically active

b. Osmotically inactive

c. Some species are osmotically active only

d. None of the above

106. Acridine dyes are more effective against:

a. Gram-positive

b. Gram-negative

c. Ricke Hsia

d. Mycoplasma

107. The mode of reproduction in Mycoplasma is:

a. Budding

b. Bursting

c. Binary fission

d. Binary fusion

108. Mycoplasmas are bacterial cells that:

a. Fail to reproduce on artificial media

b. Have a rigid cell wall

c. Are resistant to penicillin

d. Stain well with Gram stain

109. Which species is not associated with NGU?

a. *Neisseria gonorrhoeae*

b. *Mycoplasma hominis*

c. *Chlamydia trachomatis*

d. *Mycoplasma genitalium*

110. **A strain of bacteria associated with a bladder infection shows gram-negative rods. Which species is most likely to be the causative agent?**

a. *Mycoplasma hominis*

b. *Escherichia coli*

c. *Neisseria gonorrhoeae*

d. *Chlamydia trachomatis*

Answers

1.	b	31.	b	61.	b	91.	d
2.	b	32.	b	62.	c	92.	a
3.	b	33.	d	63.	c	93.	b
4.	d	34.	b	64.	d	94.	c
5.	d	35.	c	65.	d	95.	b
6.	a	36.	d	66.	a	96.	b
7.	d	37.	d	67.	a	97.	c
8.	a	38.	c	68.	d	98.	b
9.	b	39.	b	69.	d	99.	a
10.	d	40.	c	70.	c	100.	a
11.	d	41.	a	71.	b	101.	b
12.	a	42.	c	72.	b	102.	d
13.	c	43.	d	73.	b	103.	d
14.	b	44.	d	74.	b	104.	d
15.	a	45.	d	75.	c	105.	b
16.	a	46.	c	76.	b	106.	a
17.	b	47.	a	77.	b	107.	c
18.	a	48.	b	78.	b	108.	c
19.	d	49.	c	79.	a	109.	a
20.	a	50.	a	80.	d	110.	b
21.	c	51.	b	81.	c		
22.	d	52.	d	82.	a		
23.	b	53.	c	83.	a		
24.	a	54.	d	84.	d		
25.	b	55.	a	85.	c		
26.	d	56.	c	86.	d		
27.	b	57.	b	87.	d		
28.	c	58.	b	88.	d		
29.	d	59.	c	89.	d		
30.	b	60.	a	90.	d		

6 Ectoparasitic Infestation

H. Dhanalakshmi

Introduction

Entomology is the study of insects/arthropods. The word 'arthropod' is derived from the words, *arthros*, meaning jointed, and *pod*, meaning legs. Hence arthropod means 'jointed legs'. Among all living things, insects constitute the major group on Earth and play a very important role in human and animal disease transmission because they act as intermediate hosts for many diseases. They cause anaemia due to blood-sucking habit, and painful bites. The study of insects is very important for the control of many important diseases in humans and animals. This chapter covers those insects/arthropods of veterinary importance.

© CAB International 2024. *Key Questions in Preventative Farm Animal Medicine Volume 1: Types, Causes and Treatment of Infectious Diseases* (ed. T. Rana)
DOI: 10.1079/9781800624726.0006

Multiple Choice Questions

1. **The outer covering of an arthropod is called:**

   a. Chitin

   b. Chritin

   c. Skin

   d. Membrane

2. **The whole body of an insect is enclosed in:**

   a. Pupa

   b. Exoskeleton

   c. Ecdysis fluid

   d. Membrane

3. **The anterior part of the alimentary canal of an insect is called:**

   a. Stomodaeum

   b. Proctodaeum

   c. Mesodaeum

   d. Antedaeum

4. **The dorsal sclerite is also known as the:**

   a. Sternum

   b. Tergum

   c. Pleuron

   d. Lateral plate

5. **Cockroaches belong to the order:**

   a. Orthoptera

   b. Siphonoptera

   c. Diptera

   d. Coleoptera

6. **The order Mallophaga includes:**

   a. Sucking lice

   b. Biting lice

   c. Chewing lice

   d. Crab lice

7. **The antennae of lice in the order Mallophaga have:**

   a. 3–5 segments

   b. 7–8 segments

   c. 6–9 segments

   d. 1–3 segments

8. **Lice with antennae showing sexual dimorphism belong to the genus:**

   a. *Solenoptes* spp.

   b. *Hematomyzes* spp.

   c. *Columbicola* spp.

   d. *Damalinia* spp.

9. **The scientific name for shaft louse is:**

   a. *Menocanthus stramineus*

   b. *Menopon gallinae*

   c. *Menopon phaeostomum*

   d. *Trinoton anserinum*

10. **The scientific name for lice that cause 'wet feather' in ducks is:**

    a. *Menocanthus stramineus*

    b. *Menopon gallinae*

    c. *Menopon phaeostomum*

    d. *Holomenopon leucoxanthum*

11. **What is the scientific name for body louse in poultry?**

    a. *Menopon gallinae*

    b. *Menopon phaeostomum*

c. *Holomenopon leucoxanthum*

d. *Menocanthus stramineus*

12. **The louse that occurs on the least densely feathered areas of poultry is:**

a. *Menopon gallinae*

b. *Menopon phaeostomum*

c. *Holomenopon leucoxanthum*

d. *Menocanthus stramineus*

13. **Antennae are filiform in nature in lice belonging to the suborder:**

a. Amblycera

b. Ischnocera

c. Rhynchophthirina

d. Siphunculata

14. **What is the scientific name for head louse in poultry?**

a. *Lipeurus caponis*

b. *Cuclotogaster heterographus*

c. *Goniodes gigas*

d. *Goniocotes gallinae*

15. **What is the scientific name for wing louse in poultry?**

a. *Lipeurus caponis*

b. *Cuclotogaster heterographus*

c. *Goniodes gigas*

d. *Goniocotes gallinae*

16. **What is the scientific name for fluff louse in poultry?**

a. *Lipeurus caponis*

b. *Cuclotogaster heterographus*

c. *Goniodes gigas*

d. *Goniocotes gallinae*

17. **What is the scientific name for the common louse in poultry?**

    a. *Cuclogaster heterographus*

    b. *Goniocotes gallinae*

    c. *Chelopistes meleagridis*

    d. *Lipeurus caponis*

18. **What is the scientific name for short-nosed cattle louse?**

    a. *Haematopinus asini*

    b. *Haematopinus eurysternus*

    c. *Haematopinus tuberculatus*

    d. *Haematopinus bufali*

19. **Which lice occur on warthogs?**

    a. *Haematomyzus elephantis*

    b. *Haematomyzus hopkinsi*

    c. *Haematomyzus suis*

    d. *Haematomyzus caprae*

20. **Which lice are found on cats?**

    a. *Bovicola painei*

    b. *Damalinia limbata*

    c. *Trichodectes canis*

    d. *Felicola subrostratus*

21. **Sucking lice belong to the order:**

    a. Siphunculata

    b. Mallophaga

    c. Siphonoptera

    d. Hemiptera

22. **The first pair of legs are smallest in lice belonging to the family:**

    a. Linognathidae

    b. Haematopinidae

c. Menoponidae

d. Pediculidae

23. **What is the scientific name for blue louse in sheep?**

a. *Linognathus setosus*

b. *Linognathus stenopsis*

c. *Linognathus pedalis*

d. *Linognathus africanus*

24. **What is the scientific name for long-nosed cattle louse?**

a. *Linognathus setosus*

b. *Linognathus stenopsis*

c. *Linognathus vituli*

d. *Linognathus ovillus*

25. **What is the scientific name for spined rat louse?**

a. *Polyplax serrata*

b. *Hoplopleura acanthopus*

c. *Haemodipsus ventricosus*

d. *Hoploplura pacifica*

26. **The 9th abdominal segment of fleas contains the:**

a. Sensilium

b. Comb

c. Penis

d. Ovary

27. ***Spilopsyllus cuniculi* is restricted to:**

a. Rabbits

b. Cats

c. Dogs

d. Goats

28. **What is the scientific name for oriental rat flea?**

   a. *Ceratophyllus fasciatus*

   b. *Xenopsyllus cheopis*

   c. *Pulex irritans*

   d. *Ceratophyllus gallinae*

29. **What is the scientific name for black rat flea?**

   a. *Ceratophyllus fasciatus*

   b. *Xenopsyllus cheopis*

   c. *Pulex irritans*

   d. *Ceratophyllus gallinae*

30. **What is the scientific name for Jigger or chigoe flea?**

   a. *Pulex irritans*

   b. *Certophyllus columbae*

   c. *Tunga penetrans*

   d. *Pulex irritans*

31. **A hook-like structure on the last abdominal segment of a flea is called what?**

   a. Pygidium

   b. Spine

   c. Sensilium

   d. Anal strut

32. **Fleas with sharply angled frons and without ctenidia are named:**

   a. *Xenopsylla cheopis*

   b. *Echidnophaga gallinacea*

   c. *Tunga penetrans*

   d. *Pulex irritans*

33. **The frontal spine of the genal ctenidium is as long as the 2nd spine in:**

    a. *Xenopsylla cheopis*

    b. *Echidnophaga gallinacea*

    c. *Tunga penetrans*

    d. *Ctenocephalides felis*

34. **The frontal spine of the genal ctenidium is shorter than the 2nd spine in:**

    a. *Xenopsylla cheopis*

    b. *Echidnophaga gallinacea*

    c. *Tunga penetrans*

    d. *Ctenocephalides canis*

35. **The *Yersinia pestis* organism is transmitted by:**

    a. *Xenopsylla cheopis*

    b. *Echidnophaga gallinacea*

    c. *Tunga penetrans*

    d. *Ctenocephalides canis*

36. **Metamorphosis is complete in:**

    a. Lice

    b. Cockroaches

    c. Bugs

    d. Flies

37. **Antennae are longer in:**

    a. Suborder Nematocera

    b. Suborder Brachycera

    c. Suborder Cyclorrhapha

    d. Order Siphonoptera

38.   **Antennae are shorter in:**

a. Suborder Nematocera

b. Suborder Brachycera

c. Suborder Cyclorrhapha

d. Order Siphonoptera

39.   **The pupae are coarctate in:**

a. Suborder Nematocera

b. Suborder Brachycera

c. Suborder Cyclorrhapha

d. Order Siphonoptera

40.   **A ptilinal suture or frontal suture is present in flies belonging to:**

a. Suborder Nematocera

b. Suborder Brachycera

c. Suborder Cyclorrhapha

d. Order Siphonoptera

41.   **Series Schizophora comes under the suborder:**

a. Nematocera

b. Brachycera

c. Cyclorrhapha

d. Siphonoptera

42.   **Anopheles mosquitoes lay their eggs:**

a. In rafts

b. Singly

c. In groups of 5

d. In groups of 100

43. **Eggs are laid in egg rafts in the case of:**

a. *Culex*

b. *Anopheles*

c. *Culicoides*

d. *Phlebotomus*

44. ***Culicoides robertsi* causes 'Queensland itch' in**

a. Sheep

b. Cattle

c. Buffalo

d. Horses

45. ***Culicoides robertsi* causes 'sweet itch/sweat itch/summer dermatitis' in:**

a. Sheep

b. Cattle

c. Buffalo

d. Horses

46. **The common name for flies belonging to the family Simuliidae is:**

a. Buffalo gnats

b. Swarm flies

c. No-see-ums

d. Punkies

47. **The common name for flies belonging to the family Simuliidae is:**

a. Black flies

b. Swarm flies

c. No-see-ums

d. Punkies

48. **The larvae of flies having pro leg are called:**

    a. Culicoides

    b. *Simulium*

    c. Mosquitoes

    d. *Tabanus*

49. **The scientific name for potu fly is:**

    a. *Simulium indicum*

    b. *Simulium arcticum*

    c. *Simulium venustum*

    d. *Simulium callidum*

50. **Kala azar is transmitted in India by:**

    a. *Phlebotomus papatasii*

    b. *Phlebotomus argentipes*

    c. *Phlebotomus chinensis*

    d. *Phlebotomus mongolensis*

51. **The common name for Tabanus fly is:**

    a. Breeze fly

    b. No-see-ums

    c. Sweat fly

    d. Latriene fly

52. **Horseflies belong to the family:**

    a. Tabanidae

    b. Culicidae

    c. Simulidae

    d. Certopogonidae

53. **The wings of horseflies have:**

    a. Branching of cubital vein

    b. Branching of 4th longitudinal vein

c. Branching of 1st medial vein

d. Branching of 2nd longitudinal vein

54.   The proboscis is very long in which genus?

a. *Tabanus*

b. *Pangonia*

c. *Chrysops*

d. *Haematopota*

55.   The 3rd segment of the antenna of *Pangonia* has:

a. 3 annulations

b. 5 annulations

c. 4 annulations

d. 6–7 annulations

56.   The 3rd segment of the antenna has 6–7 annulations in:

a. *Tabanus*

b. *Pangonia*

c. *Chrysops*

d. *Haematopota*

57.   The 3rd segment of the antenna has 4 annulations in:

a. *Tabanus*

b. *Pangonia*

c. *Chrysops*

d. *Haematopota*

58.   Wings having a dark band passing from the anterior to the posterior border are found in:

a. *Tabanus*

b. *Pangonia*

c. *Chrysops*

d. *Haematopota*

59. **The 3rd segment of the antenna has 3 annulations in:**

a. *Tabanus*

b. *Pangonia*

c. *Chrysops*

d. *Haematopota*

60. **Wings have a characteristic mottling in:**

a. *Tabanus*

b. *Pangonia*

c. *Haematopota*

d. *Chrysops*

61. **The 3rd segment of the antenna has 4 annulations with a spur or tooth-like projection in:**

a. *Tabanus*

b. *Pangonia*

c. *Chrysops*

d. *Haematopota*

62. **Tabanid flies are very fond of:**

a. Sunlight

b. Darkness

c. Moisture

d. Wind

63. **Bots belong to the genus:**

a. *Tabanus*

b. *Gasterophilus*

c. *Musca*

d. *Stomoxys*

64. **Eggs are laid near the fetlocks of forelegs and in the scapular region by:**

   a. *Gasterophilus intestinalis*

   b. *Gasterophilus inermis*

   c. *Gasterophilus pecorum*

   d. *Gasterophilus haemorrhoidalis*

65. **Eggs are deposited on or near the cheeks by:**

   a. *Gasterophilus intestinalis*

   b. *Gasterophilus inermis*

   c. *Gasterophilus pecorum*

   d. *Gasterophilus nasalis*

66. **A closed apical cell in the wing is found in which genus?**

   a. *Tabanus*

   b. *Musca*

   c. *Stomoxys*

   d. *Chrysops*

67. **An open apical cell in the wing is found in which genus?**

   a. *Tabanus*

   b. *Musca*

   c. *Stomoxys*

   d. *Chrysops*

68. **Arista is bilaterally plumose up to the tip in which genus?**

   a. *Musca*

   b. *Stomoxys*

   c. *Haematobia*

   d. *Chrysomyia*

69. **What is the name for mouth parts adapted for imbibing liquid food?**

    a. *Musca*

    b. *Stomoxys*

    c. *Haematobia*

    d. *Chrysomyia*

70. **What is the significance of vomit drops in Musca flies?**

    a. Disease transmission

    b. Maturity phase

    c. Egg-laying phase

    d. Fly death

71. **Larvae with reduced head or no head are called:**

    a. Acephalus

    b. Eucephalus

    c. Oligopod

    d. Polypod

72. **The quiescent phase between larva and imago is the:**

    a. Adult

    b. Pupa

    c. Egg

    d. Nymph

73. **What is the name for an adult insect inside a pupa?**

    a. Imago

    b. Egg

    c. Nymph

    d. Larva

74. **The wings and legs of developing adults can be seen externally in:**

    a. Exarate pupa

    b. Obtectate pupa

c. Coarctate pupa

d. None of these

75. **Adults that emerge through a T-shaped opening in the pupal case are known as:**

a. Exarate pupa

b. Obtectate pupa

c. Coarctate pupa

d. None of these

76. **Young adults that emerge through a circular opening in the pupal case are known as:**

a. Exarate pupa

b. Obtectate pupa

c. Coarctate pupa

d. None of these

77. **An example of coarctate pupae is:**

a. House flies

b. Bedbugs

c. Tabanus

d. Ticks

78. **An example of obtectate pupae is:**

a. Mosquitoes

b. House flies

c. Bedbugs

d. Ticks

79. **An example of exarate pupae is:**

a. Bedbugs

b. Ticks

c. Beetles

d. House flies

80.   Which of the following is true about mosquitoes?

a. Male mosquitoes do not have maxillae/mandibles

b. Male mosquitoes live on blood

c. Male mosquitoes have maxillae/mandibles

d. Male mosquitoes live on flesh

81.   Wrigglers are the larvae of:

a. Ticks

b. Mites

c. Mosquitoes

d. Flies

82.   A row of spines on the ventral aspect of the siphon tube in mosquito larvae is called:

a. Comb

b. Pecten

c. Siphon

d. Gill

83.   The larvae of mosquitoes are called:

a. Wrigglers

b. Tumblers

c. a and b

d. None of these

84.   The pupae of mosquitoes are called:

a. Wrigglers

b. Tumblers

c. a and b

d. None of these

85.   A Hodge's garbage-can trap is used to catch:

a. Tabanid flies

b. Culicoides flies

c. Chrysomyia flies

d. Musca flies

86. **Which of the following is true?**

a. *Musca autumnalis* is larger than *Musca domestica*

b. *Musca autumnalis* is smaller than *Musca domestica*

c. *Musca autumnalis* is the same size as *Musca domestica*

d. *Musca autumnalis* is totally different from *Musca domestica*

87. **Use of back rubbers is indicated for the control of:**

a. Face fly

b. House fly

c. Deer fly

d. No-see-ums

88. **An example of non-metallic muscids is:**

a. *Musca domestica*

b. *Morrelia anenscens*

c. *Tabanus* spp.

d. *Stomoxys morsitrans*

89. **In the genus *Fannia*:**

a. Aristae are bare

b. Aristae are plumose

c. Aristae are plumed on one side

d. None of these

90. **Which of the following is true?**

a. *Musca domestica* is the intermediate host for the *Trypanosoma* species

b. *Musca domestica* is the intermediate host for the *Habronema* species

c. *Musca domestica* is the intermediate host for the *Dirofilaria* species

d. *Musca domestica* is the intermediate host for the *Moniezia* species

91. **Which of the following is true?**

    a. Spreading manure like slurry will control Tabanid flies

    b. Spreading manure like slurry will control Musca flies

    c. Spreading manure like slurry will control Culicoides flies

    d. Spreading manure like slurry will control mosquitoes

92. **Entomology is the study of:**

    a. Birds

    b. Animals

    c. Insects

    d. Plants

93. **Insects have:**

    a. Jointed legs

    b. Unjointed legs

    c. No legs

    d. All of these

94. **In the insect life cycle:**

    a. Pupa is the resting stage

    b. Pupa is the active phase

    c. Larva is the inactive stage

    d. Nymph is the resting stage

95. **Which insect has piercing and sucking mouth parts?**

    a. Mosquito

    b. House fly

    c. Blowfly

    d. Flesh fly

96. **Which insect has sponge-type mouth parts?**

    a. Mosquito

    b. House fly

    c. Punky

    d. Flesh fly

97. **Which insect has chewing mouth parts?**

    a. Beetle

    b. Mosquito

    c. House fly

    d. Flesh fly

98. **Which is an example of a solenophagus insect?**

    a. Mosquito

    b. Begbug

    c. Kissing bug

    d. All of these

99. **Which is an example of a telmophagus insect?**

    a. Deer fly

    b. House fly

    c. Grasshopper

    d. Flesh fly

100. **Insects that come under the order Siphonoptera include:**

    a. Lice

    b. Fleas

    c. Ticks

    d. Flies

101. **Insects that come under the class Diptera include:**

    a. Lice

    b. Fleas

c. Ticks

d. Flies

102. **Insects that come under the class Arachnida include:**

a. Lice

b. Fleas

c. Ticks

d. Flies

103. **Musca flies belong to the order:**

a. Diptera

b. Siphonoptera

c. Coleoptera

d. Hemiptera

104. **Bugs belong to the order:**

a. Diptera

b. Siphonoptera

c. Coleoptera

d. Hemiptera

105. **Complete metamorphosis is seen in:**

a. Holometabolous insects

b. Hemimetabolous insects

c. a and b

d. None of these

106. **An example of an oviparous insect would be:**

a. *Musca*

b. *Sarcophaga*

c. *Glossina*

d. *Chrysomyia*

107. **An example of a viviparous insect would be:**

a. *Musca*

b. *Sarcophaga*

c. *Glossina*

d. *Chrysomyia*

108. **Which body parts are used in the identification of fleas?**

a. Anal struts

b. Genal combs

c. Legs

d. Abdominal segments

109. **Insects breathe through their:**

a. Lungs

b. Gills

c. Nostrils

d. Spiracles

110. **Respiratory spiracles are always located on the:**

a. Sternum

b. Tergum

c. Pleuron

d. Notum

111. **The scientific name for relapsing fever tick is:**

a. *Ornithodoros moubata*

b. *Ornithodoros savignyi*

c. *Ornithodoros turicata*

d. *Ornithodoros parkeri*

112. **A tampan which has an eye is:**

a. *Ornithodoros moubata*

b. *Ornithodoros savignyi*

c. a and b

d. None of these

113. **The common name for *Fannia scalaris* is:**

a. Latrine fly

b. Fruit fly

c. Face fly

d. House fly

114. **The tertiary striker in blow fly strike is:**

a. *Fannia scalaris*

b. *Fannia australis*

c. *Fannia canicularis*

d. *Fannia benjamini*

115. **The scientific name for stable fly is:**

a. *Musca domestica*

b. *Stomoxys calcitrans*

c. *Fannia scalaris*

d. *Morrelia simplex*

116. **The scientific name for eyeless tampan is:**

a. *Argas persicus*

b. *Argas rerlexus*

c. *Ornithodoros moubata*

d. *Argas reflexus*

117. **The scientific name for sheep head fly is:**

a. *Stomoxys calcitrans*

b. *Hydrotaea irritans*

c. *Hydrotaea occulta*

d. *Musca domestica*

118. **Which of the following is true?**

    a. *Hydrotaea irritans* resembles a house fly

    b. *Stomoxys calcitrans* resembles a house fly

    c. *Morrelia simplex* resembles a house fly

    d. None of these

119. **The aristae are haired on the dorsal surface only in:**

    a. Genus *Musca*

    b. Genus *Stomoxys*

    c. Genus *Haematobia*

    d. Genus *Hydrotaea*

120. **The scientific name for Indian buffalo fly is:**

    a. *Haematobia exigua*

    b. *Haematobia minuta*

    c. *Haematobia stimulans*

    d. *Haematobia irritans*

121. **The scientific name for horn fly is:**

    a. *Haematobia exigua*

    b. *Haematobia minuta*

    c. *Haematobia stimulans*

    d. *Haematobia irritans*

122. **The scientific name for tsetse fly is:**

    a. *Glossina*

    b. *Tabanus*

    c. *Phlebotomus*

    d. *Culicoides*

123. **The wing has hatchet-shaped discal cells in which genus?**

    a. *Musca*

    b. *Glossina*

   c. *Stomoxys*

   d. *Haematobia*

124. **A chequerboard-marked abdomen is seen in:**

   a. Flesh flies

   b. Fruit flies

   c. House flies

   d. Horn flies

125. **The chief cause of blowfly strike in sheep in Australia is:**

   a. *Lucilia sericata*

   b. *Lucilia cuprina*

   c. *Lucilia caesar*

   d. *Lucilia illustris*

126. **The scientific name for green bottle flies is:**

   a. *Lucilia*

   b. *Calliphora*

   c. *Chrysomyia*

   d. *Phormia*

127. **The scientific name for copper bottle flies is:**

   a. *Calliphora*

   b. *Lucilia*

   c. *Chrysomyia*

   d. *Phormia*

128. **The scientific name for blue bottle flies is:**

   a. *Lucilia*

   b. *Calliphora*

   c. *Chrysomyia*

   d. *Phormia*

129. **The scientific name for black blow flies is:**

    a. *Lucilia*

    b. *Calliphora*

    c. *Chrysomyia*

    d. *Phormia*

130. **The scientific name for bluish-green flies is:**

    a. *Lucilia*

    b. *Calliphora*

    c. *Chrysomyia*

    d. *Phormia*

131. **The scientific name for old world screwworm fly is:**

    a. *Chrysomyia chloropya*

    b. *Chrysomyia albiceps*

    c. *Chrysomyia micropogon*

    d. *Chrysomyia bezziana*

132. **Calliphorine myiasis is commonly known as:**

    a. Black myiasis

    b. Strike

    c. Blue strike

    d. None of these

133. **Myiasis in the dorsal region of the body is called:**

    a. Body strike

    b. Poll strike

    c. Pizzle strike

    d. Breech strike

134. **The chemical used for the control of pizzle strike is:**

    a. 40% phenol

    b. 40% formalin

c. 20% phenol

d. 20% formalin

135. **'Mule's operation' is an older surgical technique for the control of:**

a. Blow fly strike

b. Tabanus fly bite

c. Culicoides fly attack

d. None of these

136. **'Crutching' is a term for:**

a. Clipping the wool from the tail region

b. Clipping the wool from the head region

c. Clipping the wool around a wound region

d. Clipping the wool from the facial region

137. **Screwworm is the name given to the larvae of:**

a. *Callitroga hominivorax*

b. *Chrysomyia bezziana*

c. *Cordylobia anthropophaga*

d. None of these

138. **The scientific name for tumbu fly is:**

a. *Callitroga hominivorax*

b. *Chrysomyia bezziana*

c. *Cordylobia anthropophaga*

d. None of these

139. **The scientific name for skin maggot fly is:**

a. *Callitroga hominivorax*

b. *Chrysomyia bezziana*

c. *Cordylobia anthropophaga*

d. None of these

140. **The scientific name for Lund's fly is:**

    a. *Cordylobia rodhaini*

    b. *Cordylobia anthropophaga*

    c. *Callitroga hominivorax*

    d. *Chrysomyia bezziana*

141. **The scientific name for foot maggot fly is:**

    a. *Cordylobia rodhaini*

    b. *Cordylobia anthropophaga*

    c. *Booponus intonsus*

    d. *Chrysomyia bezziana*

142. **The scientific name for Congo floor maggot fly is:**

    a. *Booponus intonsus*

    b. *Cordylobia rodhaini*

    c. *Auchmeromyia luteola*

    d. *Pollenia rudis*

143. **The larvae of *Pollenia rudis* are seen in:**

    a. Beetles

    b. Fruit

    c. Ants

    d. Earthworms

144. **The common name for *Sarcophaga* fly is:**

    a. Fruit fly

    b. Flesh fly

    c. Maggot fly

    d. Latriene fly

145. **The common name for *Wohlfahrtia magnifica* is:**

    a. Screwworm fly

    b. Flesh fly

    c. Old world screwworm fly

    d. Old world flesh fly

146.   **The common name for *Oestrus ovis* is:**

    a. Sheep nasal fly

    b. Fruit fly

    c. Horse bot fly

    d. None of these

147.   **False gid in sheep is produced by:**

    a. *Oestrus ovis*

    b. *Coenurus ovis*

    c. *Coenurus cerebralis*

    d. None of the above

148.   ***Rhinoestrus purpurensis* is found in the nasal sinuses of:**

    a. Sheep

    b. Goats

    c. Horses

    d. Pigs

149.   **The scientific name for camel nasal bot fly is:**

    a. *Cephalopsis titillator*

    b. *Oestrus ovis*

    c. *Rhinoestrus purpurensis*

    d. *Cochliomyia hominivorax*

150.   **The scientific name for elephant throat bot fly is:**

    a. *Oestrus ovis*

    b. *Rhinoestrus purpurensis*

    c. *Cochliomyia hominivorax*

    d. *Pharyngobolus africanus*

151. **The scientific name for northern cattle grub is:**

    a. *Hypoderma bovis*

    b. *Hypoderma lineatum*

    c. *Hypoderma ovis*

    d. *Hypoderma caprae*

152. **The scientific name for common cattle grub is:**

    a. *Hypoderma bovis*

    b. *Hypoderma lineatum*

    c. *Hypoderma ovis*

    d. *Hypoderma caprae*

153. **The scientific name for common heel fly is:**

    a. *Hypoderma bovis*

    b. *Hypoderma lineatum*

    c. *Hypoderma ovis*

    d. *Hypoderma caprae*

154. **Which of the following flies lays single eggs?**

    a. *Oestrus ovis*

    b. *Hypoderma bovis*

    c. *Hypoderma lineatum*

    d. *Cephalopsis titilator*

155. **Which of the following flies lays its eggs in rows of six or more?**

    a. *Oestrus ovis*

    b. *Hypoderma bovis*

    c. *Hypoderma lineatum*

    d. *Pharyngobolus africanus*

156. **Larvae of *Hypoderma diana* occur in:**

    a. Deer

    b. Cattle

c. Sheep

d. Horses

157. *Hypoderma ageratum* **larvae occur in:**

a. Deer

b. Cattle

c. Sheep

d. Horses

158. *Hypoderma crossi* **is seen in India on:**

a. Cattle and buffalo

b. Horses and donkeys

c. Sheep and goats

d. Humans

159. **Berne in man is due to:**

a. *Dermatobia hominis*

b. *Hypoderma diana*

c. *Oestrus ovis*

d. *Hypoderma bovis*

160. **Nuche in man is due to:**

a. *Cephalopsis titilator*

b. *Dermatobia hominis*

c. *Hypoderma ovis*

d. *Hypoderma bovis*

161. **Forcel in man is due to:**

a. *Cephalopsis titilator*

b. *Dermatobia hominis*

c. *Hypoderma ovis*

d. *Hypoderma bovis*

162. *Cuterebra emasculator* causes:

   a. Parasitic castration

   b. Parasitic sinusitis

   c. Parasitic gastritis

   d. Parasitic hair loss

163. **Pupiparan flies give birth to:**

   a. Larvae

   b. Pupae

   c. Eggs

   d. Larvae ready to pupate

164. **The family that includes forest flies is the:**

   a. Oestridae

   b. Simuliidae

   c. Sarcophagidae

   d. Hippoboscidae

165. **Hippobosca flies transmit:**

   a. *Babesia bovis*

   b. *Theileria annulata*

   c. *Trypanosoma theileri*

   d. None of these

166. **Hippoboscid fly, mainly found on dogs, is:**

   a. *Hippobosca equine*

   b. *Hippobosca capensis*

   c. *Hippobosca camelina*

   d. *Hippobosca macualata*

167. **The scientific name for sheep ked is:**

   a. *Oestrus ovis*

   b. *Melophagus ovinus*

c. *Hippobosca capensis*

d. *Chrysomyia bezziana*

168. **Trypanosoma malophagium is transmitted by:**

a. Nasal bot fly

b. Sheep ked

c. Buffalo fly

d. Horn fly

169. **Haemoproteus columbae is transmitted by:**

a. *Pseudolynchia canariensis*

b. *Melophagus ovinus*

c. *Columbicola columbae*

d. None of these

170. **Flies that cast off their wings when they find a host belong to the genus:**

a. *Hippobosca*

b. *Lipoptena*

c. *Pseudolynchia*

d. *Melophagus*

171. **In arachnids, the term 'prosoma' refers to:**

a. The 1st 2 segments of the body

b. The 1st 6 segments of the body

c. The 1st segment of the body

d. None of these

172. **In arachnids, the term 'opisthosoma' refers to:**

a. The 1st 2 segments of the body

b. The 1st 6 segments of the body

c. The 1st segment of the body

d. None of these

173. **Prosoma bears:**

a. Chelicerae

b. Pedipalps

c. Four pairs of walking legs

d. All of these

174. **Opisthosoma bears:**

a. Chelicerae

b. Pedipalps

c. Four pairs of walking legs

d. All of these

175. **Prosoma is divided into:**

a. Gnathosoma and podosoma

b. Head and abdomen

c. Head only

d. Thorax and abdomen

176. **Podosoma and Opisthosoma are together known as:**

a. Idiosoma

b. Gnathosoma

c. Prosoma

d. None of these

177. **Gnathosoma bears:**

a. Only Chelicerae

b. Chelicerae and pedipalps

c. Only pedipalps

d. Only legs

178. **Gnathosoma of ticks and mites is called:**

a. Gnathobases

b. Capitulum

c. Chelicerae

d. Pedipalps

179.   A tooth-like structure on the gnathosoma is called a:

a. Pedipalp

b. Chelicerae

c. Hypostome

d. Capitulum

180.   *Dermanyssus gallinae* is also known as:

a. Red mite of poultry

b. Northern mite of poultry

c. Southern mite of poultry

d. None of these

181.   *Dermanyssus gallinae* transmits:

a. *Trypanosoma brucei*

b. *Plasmodium relictum*

c. *Haemoproteus columbae*

d. *Borrelia anserina*

182.   *Ornithonyssus sylviarum* is also known as:

a. Red mite of poultry

b. Northern mite of poultry

c. Southern mite of poultry

d. None of these

183.   *Ornithonyssus bursa* is commonly known as:

a. Red mite of poultry

b. Northern mite of poultry

c. Tropical fowl mite

d. Tropical rat mite

184. ***Ornithonyssus bacoti* is commonly known as:**

    a. Red mite of poultry

    b. Northern mite of poultry

    c. Tropical fowl mite

    d. Tropical rat mite

185. ***Allodermanyssus sanguineus* is commonly known as:**

    a. Red mite of poultry

    b. Northern mite of poultry

    c. House mouse mite

    d. Tropical rat mite

186. **Which mite infests the nasal passage and nasal sinuses?**

    a. *Pneumonyssus caninum*

    b. *Pneumonyssus simicola*

    c. *Allodermanyssus sanguineus*

    d. *Ornithonyssus bursa*

187. **Which mite infests the bronchi?**

    a. *Pneumonyssus caninum*

    b. *Pneumonyssus simicola*

    c. *Allodermanyssus sanguineus*

    d. *Ornithonyssus bursa*

188. **The scientific name for spinose ear tick is:**

    a. *Argas persicus*

    b. *Otobius megnini*

    c. *Ornithodoros moubata*

    d. *Argas reflexus*

189. **The scientific name for castor bean tick is:**

    a. *Ixodes ricinus*

    b. *Ixodes persulcatus*

c. *Ixodes rubicundus*

d. *Ixodes canisuga*

190. **The scientific name for shoulder tick is:**

a. *Ixodes scapularis*

b. *Ixodes persulcatus*

c. *Ixodes rubicundus*

d. *Ixodes canisuga*

191. **The scientific name for black-legged tick is:**

a. *Ixodes scapularis*

b. *Ixodes persulcatus*

c. *Ixodes pilosus*

d. *Ixodes canisuga*

192. **The scientific name for North American tick is:**

a. *Boophilus microplus*

b. *Boophilus annulatus*

c. *Boophilus decoloratus*

d. None of these

193. **The scientific name for blue tick is:**

a. *Boophilus microplus*

b. *Boophilus annulatus*

c. *Boophilus decoloratus*

d. None of these

194. **The scientific name for brown ear tick is:**

a. *Rhipicephalus appendiculatus*

b. *Rhipicephalus capensis*

c. *Rhipicephalus sanguineus*

d. *Rhipicephalus evertsi*

195. The scientific name for yellow dog tick is:

a. *Haemaphysalis leachi leachi*

b. *Haemaphysalis leporis*

c. *Haemaphysalis longicornis*

d. *Haemaphysalis humerosa*

196. The scientific name for rabbit tick is:

a. *Haemaphysalis leachi leachi*

b. *Haemaphysalis leporis*

c. *Haemaphysalis longicornis*

d. *Haemaphysalis humerosa*

197. The scientific name for bush tick is:

a. *Haemaphysalis leachi leachi*

b. *Haemaphysalis leporis*

c. *Haemaphysalis longicornis*

d. *Haemaphysalis humerosa*

198. The scientific name for Rocky mountain wood tick is:

a. *Dermacentor reticulatus*

b. *Dermacentor marginatus*

c. *Dermacentor andersoni*

d. *Dermacentor variabilis*

199. The scientific name for American dog tick is:

a. *Dermacentor reticulatus*

b. *Dermacentor marginatus*

c. *Dermacentor andersoni*

d. *Dermacentor variabilis*

200. The common name for *Dermacentor nitens* is:

a. Tropical horse tick

b. Moose tick

c. Pacific coast tick

d. Brown winter tick

201. The common name for *Dermacentor albipictus* is:

a. Tropical horse tick

b. Moose tick

c. Pacific coast tick

d. Brown winter tick

202. The scientific name for bont tick is:

a. *Amblyomma hebraeum*

b. *Amblyomma variegatum*

c. *Amblyomma americanum*

d. *Amblyomma maculatum*

203. The scientific name for lone star tick is:

a. *Amblyomma hebraeum*

b. *Amblyomma variegatum*

c. *Amblyomma americanum*

d. *Amblyomma maculatum*

204. The scientific name for Gulf Coast tick is:

a. *Amblyomma hebraeum*

b. *Amblyomma variegatum*

c. *Amblyomma americanum*

d. *Amblyomma maculatum*

205. *Trombicula autumnalis* is also called:

a. Harvest mite

b. Sterile mite

c. Burrowing mite

d. Follicle mite

206. **A 'mousy' odour occurs in infections due to:**

    a. Harvest mite

    b. Follicular mite

    c. Chigger mite

    d. Burrowing mite

207. **Australian itch mite belongs to the genus:**

    a. *Demodex*

    b. *Sarcoptes*

    c. *Psorergates*

    d. *Cheyletiella*

208. **Rabbit fur mite belongs to the genus:**

    a. *Demodex*

    b. *Sarcoptes*

    c. *Psorergates*

    d. *Cheyletiella*

209. **Which is true?**

    a. Sarcoptic mange in horses is a notifiable disease

    b. Demodicosis in man is a notifiable disease

    c. Demodicosis in cattle is a notifiable disease

    d. None of these

210. ***Cnemidocoptes mutans* causes:**

    a. Scaly leg in birds

    b. Scab in sheep

    c. Depluming itch in birds

    d. Itching in dogs

211. ***Psoroptes ovis* causes:**

    a. Scaly leg in birds

    b. Scab in sheep

c. Depluming itch in birds

d. Itching in dogs

212. ***Chorioptes bovis* causes:**

a. Scaly leg in birds

b. Scab in sheep

c. Depluming itch in birds

d. Itchy legs in cattle

Answers

1.	a	31.	d	62.	a	93.	a
2.	b	32.	b	63.	b	94.	a
3.	a	33.	d	64.	a	95.	a
4.	a	34.	d	65.	b	96.	b
5.	a	35.	a	66.	b	97.	a
6.	a	36.	d	67.	c	98.	d
7.	a	37.	a	68.	a	99.	a
8.	c	38.	b	69.	a	100.	b
9.	b	39.	c	70.	a	101.	d
10.	d	40.	c	71.	a	102.	c
11.	d	41.	c	72.	b	103.	a
12.	d	42.	b	73.	a	104.	d
13.	b	43.	a	74.	a	105.	a
14.	b	44.	d	75.	b	106.	a
15.	a	45.	d	76.	c	107.	c
16.	d	46.	a	77.	a	108.	b
17.	c	47.	a	78.	a	109.	d
18.	b	48.	b	79.	c	110.	b
19.	b	49.	a	80.	a	111.	c
20.	d	50.	b	81.	c	112.	b
21.	a	51.	a	82.	b	113.	a
22.	a	52.	a	83.	a	114.	b
23.	d	53.	b	84.	b	115.	b
23.	c	54.	b	85.	d	116.	c
24.	c	55.	d	86.	a	117.	b
25.	a	56.	b	87.	a	118.	a
26.	a	57.	c	88.	b	119.	c
27.	a	58.	d	89.	a	120.	a
28.	b	59.	d	90.	b	121.	d
29.	b	60.	c	91.	b	122.	a
30.	c	61.	a	92.	c	123.	b

(Continued)

124.	a	147.	a	170.	b	193.	c
125.	b	148.	c	171.	b	194.	a
126.	a	149.	a	172.	d	195.	a
127.	b	150.	d	173.	a	196.	b
128.	b	151.	a	174.	c	197.	c
129.	d	152.	b	175.	a	198.	c
130.	c	153.	b	176.	a	199.	d
131.	d	154.	b	177.	b	200.	a
132.	b	155.	c	178.	b	201.	b
133.	a	156.	a	179.	c	202.	a
134.	a	157.	c	180.	a	203.	c
135.	a	158.	a	181.	d	204.	d
136.	a	159.	a	182.	b	205.	a
137.	a	160.	b	183.	c	206.	b
138.	c	161.	b	184.	d	207.	c
139.	c	162.	a	185.	c	208.	d
140.	a	163.	d	186.	a	209.	a
141.	c	164.	d	187.	b	210.	a
142.	c	165.	c	188.	a	211.	b
143.	d	166.	b	189.	a	212.	d
144.	b	167.	b	190.	a		
145.	d	168.	b	191.	a		
146.	a	169.	a	192.	b		

7 Endoparasitic Infections

Bhupamani Das and Sivajothi Srigireddy

Introduction

Helminth (parasitic worm) infections of domestic animals are a major constraint on efficient livestock production (Charlier *et al.,* 2014). The effect of the infection is determined by a combination of factors, of which the varying susceptibility of the host species, the pathogenicity of the parasite species, the host/parasite interaction and the infective dose are the most important. Economic losses are closely associated with the extent to which the pathogenic effect of helminth infections influences the production of the individual host. This may vary considerably, from clinical disease (including mortality) to chronic production losses which may appear as reduced growth rate, weight loss or reduced fecundity. Or it may go completely unnoticed. The transmission success of the majority of economically important helminth infections of animals depends almost entirely upon ingestion of the parasites via certain food elements. Thus, herbivorous and carnivorous hosts become infected by the consumption of fodder contaminated with infective larvae and the continuation of the parasites' life cycles is secured by the host disseminating pre-infective stages onto the pasture or other food items.

Direct host-to-host transfer in helminth infections is restricted to a few parasites where prenatal infections from the mother to the growing embryo may occur and to transmission via skin penetration. Some of the filarial worms are transmitted by vector, some trematodes, like *Fasciola gigantica* by aquatic snails, whereas cestodes like *Moniezia* spp. are transmitted by oribatid mite. In addition to the helminth infections which cause direct economic losses due to reduced animal production, yet another dimension is added by the fact that several helminth infections can be transmitted to humans (zoonoses).

Successful control of helminth diseases is highly dependent on available information about local conditions and the strength of the extension

© CAB International 2024. *Key Questions in Preventative Farm Animal Medicine*
Volume 1: Types, Causes and Treatment of Infectious Diseases (ed. T. Rana)
DOI: 10.1079/9781800624726.0007

service transferring this knowledge to the farmer. Anthelmintics have been used for many years to treat clinical outbreaks of endoparasitic disease in different animals. With the advent of modern drugs that are both broader in spectrum and much less toxic than many of the early compounds, large-scale prophylactic use of anthelmintics has been possible. This may lead to the problem of resistance (Marriner and Armour, 1986). The degree and extent of this problem, especially with respect to multidrug resistance in nematode populations, has been growing. Maintaining parasites in refugia and not exposed to anthelmintics seems to be a key strategy in controlling and delaying the development of resistance, because susceptible genes are preserved. Additionally, adoption of strict quarantine measures and a combination drug strategy are two important methods for preventing anthelmintic resistance. It has also been suggested that control schemes should not rely on the sole use of anthelmintics, but employ other more complex and sustainable solutions, including parasite-resistant breeds, nutrition, pasture management, nematode-trapping fungi, antiparasitic vaccines and botanical dewormers (Shalaby, 2013).

References

Charlier, J., van der Voort, M., Kenyon, F., Skuce, P. and Vercruysse, J. (2014) Chasing helminths and their economic impact on farmed ruminants. *Trends in Parasitology* 30(7), 361–367. https://doi.org/10.1016/j.pt.2014.04.009

Marriner, S. and Armour, J. (1986) Nematode infections of domestic animals: gastrointestinal infections. In: Campbell, W.C. and Rew, R.S. (eds) *Chemotherapy of Parasitic Diseases*. Springer, Boston, MA. https://doi.org/10.1007/978-1-4684-1233-8_14

Shalaby, H. (2013) Anthelmintics resistance: How to overcome it? *Iranian journal of Parasitology* 8, 18–32.

Multiple Choice Questions

1. **Clay-pipe cirrhosis in cattle occurs due to:**

   a. Fasciolosis

   b. Monieziosis

   c. Paramphistomosis

   d. Schistosomosis

2. **One of the biological control measures of snails is:**

   a. Mechanical collection of snails

   b. Planting of poisonous trees

   c. Rearing of fish in water

   d. Applying chemicals on pastures and water

3. **Fasciolosis affected animals are prone to:**

   a. Listeriosis

   b. Salmonellosis

   c. Tuberculosis

   d. All of these

4. **The dose rate of triclabendazole for treatment of liver fluke infection in cattle and buffalo is:**

   a. 5–10 mg/kg BWT

   b. 10–12 mg/kg BWT

   c. 15–25 mg/kg BWT

   d. 25–50 mg/kg BWT

5. **Slime balls are observed in the lifecycle of:**

   a. *Fasciola hepatica*

   b. *Gastrothylax crumenifer*

   c. *Dicrocelum dendriticum*

   d. *Fasciolopsis buski*

6. **A unisexual trematode is:**

    a. Liver fluke

    b. Ruminal fluke

    c. Blood fluke

    d. Oviduct fluke

7. **The drug of choice against immature amphistomosis is:**

    a. Anthiomaline

    b. Oxyclozanide

    c. Piperazine citrate

    d. Proziquantel

8. **The longevity of metacercariae of *Fasciola* sp. under labora-tory conditions is**

    a. More than 1 hour

    b. More than 1 day

    c. More than 1 month

    d. More than 1 year

9. **The location of *Gigantocotyle explanatum* in buffalo is:**

    a. Lung

    b. Bile duct

    c. Large intestine

    d. Rumen

10. **Which is a commonly used chemical to control snails?**

    a. NaCl

    b. NaOH

    c. KOH

    d. $CuSO_4$

11. **Cercarial dermatitis is associated with:**

    a. Amphistomes

    b. Lung flukes

    c. Schistosomes

    d. Lung worms

12. **In the lifecycle of *Schistosoma nasale*, the following stage is absent:**

    a. Egg

    b. Miracidia

    c. Redia

    d. Cercaria

13. **What shape is the egg in *Schistosoma nasalis*?**

    a. Spindle

    b. Boomerang shaped

    c. Oval

    d. Elongated

14. **Which is a free-living larval stage of trematodes?**

    a. Sporocyst

    b. Miracidium

    c. Redia

    d. Daughter sporocyct

15. **Which is the definitive host of *Fasciolopsis buski*?**

    a. Sheep and goats

    b. Cattle

    c. Pigs and man

    d. Horses

16. **What is the name for 'coffee-seed' parasites occurring in pairs within lung cysts?**

    a. *Opistorchis tenuicollis*

    b. *Stephanurus dentatus*

    c. *Ascaridia galli*

    d. *Paragonimus westermanii*

17. **Which of the following is employed in the biological control of *Schistosoma* larvae?**

    a. *Heterophyes*

    b. *Platynosomum*

    c. *Chlonorchis*

    d. *Eurytrema*

18. **The common mode of infection in *Schistosoma nasale* is by:**

    a. Oral route

    b. Skin penetration

    c. Ingestion of snails

    d. Auto infection

19. **The trematode present in the mesenteric vein of cattle is:**

    a. *Fasciola hepatica*

    b. *Fasciola gigantica*

    c. *Schistosoma spindale*

    d. *Paramphistomum cervi*

20. **Which of these has a 'Napoleon hat'-shaped egg with a spine?**

    a. *Schistosoma spindale*

    b. *Schistosoma indicum*

    c. *Schistosoma nasale*

    d. *Spirocerca lupi*

21. **Black disease is associated with:**

    a. *Fasciola* spp.

    b. *Heterkis* spp.

    c. *Ornithobilharzia* spp.

    d. *Cotylophoron* spp.

22. **The definitive host of *Fasciolopsis buski* is:**

    a. Sheep

    b. Fowl

    c. Pigs and man

    d. Horses

23. ***Paragonimus westermanii* is commonly known as:**

    a. Lancet fluke

    b. Rumen fluke

    c. Lung fluke

    d. Blood fluke

24. **The snail, *Bithynia leachi*, and several fish are the intermediate hosts for:**

    a. *Cotylophoron* spp.

    b. *Schistosoma* spp.

    c. *Fasciola* spp.

    d. *Opisthorchis* spp.

25. **Which tumour causes fluke?**

    a. *Gigantocotyle explanatum*

    b. *Fasciolopsis buski*

    c. *Opisthorchis tenuicollis*

    d. *Dicrocoelium dendriticum*

26. **An amphistome is found in the bile duct of:**

    a. *Gastrothylax crumenifer*

    b. *Gigantocotyle explanatum*

c. *Paramphistomum cervi*

d. *Cotylophoron cotylophorum*

27. **The infective stage of a trematode is:**

a. Miracidium

b. 3rd stage larva

c. Sporocyst

d. Metacercaria

28. **Soft-shelled or shell-less eggs are laid by hens infected with:**

a. *Cotugnia digonopora*

b. *Syngamus trache*

c. *Heterakis gallinarum*

d. *Prosthogonimus ovatus*

29. **Ingestion of raw or improperly cooked fish can lead to which infection?**

a. *Fasciolopsis buski*

b. *Dicrocoelium dendriticum*

c. *Opisthorchis tenuicollis*

d. *Paragonimus westermanii*

30. **The eggs of *Schistosoma indicum* are:**

a. Oval shaped

b. Spindle shaped

c. Boomerang shaped

d. Triangular shaped

31. **Which among the following is a larval stage of a trematode?**

a. Cysticercus

b. Hydatid

c. Cercaria

d. Coenurus

32. **Identify the equine amphistome from the following:**

    a. *Paramphistomum*

    b. *Gigantocotyle*

    c. *Gastrodiscus*

    d. *Gastrothylax*

33. **All five larval stages are present in the life cycle of:**

    a. *Cotylophoron*

    b. *Schistosoma*

    c. *Dicrocoelium*

    d. *Prosthogonimus*

34. **Name the largest helminth egg from the following:**

    a. Egg of amphistome

    b. Egg of *Moniezia*

    c. Egg of *Toxocara*

    d. Egg of *Strongyloides*

35. **The infective stage of a trematode is:**

    a. Miracidium

    b. 3rd-stage larva

    c. Sporocyst

    d. Metacercaria

36. **Which is the smallest tapeworm in poultry?**

    a. *Railleitina cesticellus*

    b. *Railleitina tatragona*

    c. *Echinococcus granulosus*

    d. *Daveinea proglottina*

37. **'Measly beef' is associated with:**

    a. *Cysticercus cellulosae*

    b. *Cysticercus bovis*

   c. *Coenurus cerebralis*

   d. *Cysticercus taenuicollis*

38. **In *Dipyllidium caninum*, the segments resemble:**

   a. Ragiseed

   b. Cucumber seed

   c. Cooked rice

   d. Beans

39. ***Dipyllobothrium latum* infection leads to deficiency of:**

   a. Vitamin B

   b. Vitamin B12

   c. Vitamin D

   d. Vitamin C

40. **The location of *Moniezia expansa* is:**

   a. Small intestine of sheep

   b. Abamasum of sheep

   c. Caecum of horses

   d. Large intestine of dogs

41. **A cestode bearing lappets behind the sucker is a characteristic feature of:**

   a. *Moniezia expansa*

   b. *Anaplocephala perifoliata*

   c. *Paranoplocephala mammillana*

   d. *Avitellina centripunctata*

42. ***Coenurus cerebralis* develops in the:**

   a. Brain and spinal cord of sheep

   b. Brain and spinal cord of cattle

   c. Brain and spinal cord of pigs

   d. Brain and spinal cord of dogs

43. **A metacestode with a single non-invaginated scolex drawn into a small vesicle without a cavity is called a:**

a. Cysticercus

b. Cysticercoid

c. Coenurus

d. Hydatid

44. **The location of *Davaina proglottina* in fowl is:**

a. Gizzard

b. Crop

c. Deuodenum

d. Oesophagus

45. **The larval form of *T. solium* is:**

a. *Cysticercus cellulosae*

b. *Cysticercus bovis*

c. *Cysticercus taenicollis*

d. *Coenurus cerebralis*

46. **Acanthocephalids are commonly known as:**

a. Blood flukes

b. Ruminal flukes

c. Thorny-headed worms

d. Oviduct flukes

47. **In *Echinococcus granulosus*, the infective stage is:**

a. Cystacanth

b. Hexacanth egg

c. Quadrinucleated cyst

d. Sporulated oocyst

48. **The infective stage of *Moniezia expansa* is:**

a. Cysticercus

b. Coenurus

c. Cysticercoid

d. Tetrathyridium

49. **Neurocysticercosis is associated with:**

a. *Taenia solium*

b. *Taenia saginata*

c. *Taenia multiceps*

d. *Taenia hydatigena*

50. **Nodular taeniasis is caused by:**

a. *Taenia solium*

b. *Taenia taeniaformis*

c. *Raillietina echinobothridia*

d. *Echinococcus granulosus*

51. **The eggs of which of these have a 'cartwheel' appearance?**

a. *Taenia spp.*

b. *Cotylophoron cotylophorum*

c. *Toxocara canis*

d. *Ascaris suum*

52. **Which of these has a 'cooked rice grain'-shaped gravid segment?**

a. *Taenia* spp.

b. *Moniezia* spp.

c. *Diphylidium caninum*

d. *Choanotaenia infundibulum*

53. **The larval cestode present in the lungs and liver of sheep is:**

a. *Cysticercus bovis*

b. Hydatid cyst

c. Tetrathyridium

d. Larvae of *Dictyocaulus filaria*

54. **Anal pruritus in dogs is produced by:**

a. *Oxyuris equi*

b. *Enterobius* spp.

c. *Dipylidium caninum*

d. *Toxocara canis*

55. **The cestode present in the ileo-caecal junction of horses is:**

a. *Moniezia* spp.

b. *Fascioloides magna*

c. *Davainea proglottina*

d. *Anoplocephala perfoliata*

56. **The intermediate host of *Taenia saginata* is:**

a. Rats

b. Rabbits

c. Cattle

d. Sheep

57. **Egg pockets are commonly observed in the gravid segments of:**

a. *Hymenolepis carioca*

b. *Diphllobothrium latum*

c. *Davainea proglottina*

d. *Dypylidium caninum*

58. **Inter-proglottidal glands are present in:**

a. *Avitellina* spp.

b. *Anaplocephala* spp.

c. *Moniezia* spp.

d. *Taenia* spp.

59. **The smallest tapeworm in dogs is:**

a. *Dipylidium caninum*

b. *Taenia multiceps*

c. *Taenia hydatigena*

d. *Echinococcus granulosus*

60. **Diagnosis of cestode infection in poultry is made by looking for:**

a. Eggs in the dropping

b. Larvae

c. Gravid segments

d. Cysticercus

61. **Dipyllidiosis in dogs can be controlled by killing:**

a. Mosquitoes

b. Flies

c. Fleas

d. Bugs

62. **Eggs with a hexacanth embryo are seen in:**

a. Roundworms

b. Tapeworms

c. Flukes

d. Insects

63. **Which translucent metacestode has groups of invaginated scolecies on the germinal layer?**

a. Cysticercus

b. Hydatid cyst

c. Cysticercoid

d. Coenurus

64. **The infective stage of larvae in cotyloda is known as:**

a. Pleurocercoid

b. Procercoid

c. Coracidium

d. All of these

65.   **A hydatid cyst is the larval form of:**

   a. *Moniezia* spp.

   b. *Multiceps* spp.

   c. *Taenia* spp.

   d. *Echinococcus* spp.

66.   **Ingestion of *Ctenocephalides canis, Trichodectis canis* can transmit:**

   a. *Dipylidium* spp.

   b. *Amoebotaenia* spp.

   c. *Railliettina* spp.

   d. *Taenia* spp.

67.   **Metameric segmentation of the body is seen in:**

   a. Trematodes

   b. Cestodes

   c. Nematodes

   d. Acanthocephala

68.   **The larval stage of poultry tapeworm is:**

   a. Procercoid

   b. Plerocercoid

   c. Cysticercoid

   d. Cysticercus

69.   **The dwarf tapeworm seen in equines is:**

   a. *Anoplocephala perfolita*

   b. *Davainea proglottina*

   c. *Amoebotaenia cuneata*

   d. *Paranoplocepha mamillana*

70. **Lambs infected with *Moniezia* spp. are predisposed to:**

a. Enterotoxaemia

b. Black disease

c. Black quarter

d. Johne's disease

71. **Which cestode causes nodules in the small intestine of sheep?**

a. *Moniezia benedeni*

b. *Diphyllobothrium latum*

c. *Stilesia globipunctata*

d. *Avitellina lahorea*

72. **Each egg packet of *Dipylidium caninum* contains:**

a. 12 eggs

b. 6 eggs

c. 30 eggs

d. 15 eggs

73. **Gid in sheep is caused by:**

a. Hydatid cyst

b. *Cysticercus tenuicollis*

c. Cysticercoid

d. *Coenurus cerebralis*

74. **The organs of attachment in cotyloda are:**

a. Suckers

b. Bothrida

c. Bothria

d. Hooks

75. **Regularly alternating genital openings are present in:**

a. *Dipylidium* spp.

b. *Hymenolepis* spp.

c. *Taenia* spp.

d. *Davainea* spp.

76. **Cysticercus is a larval stage which occurs in the life cycle of:**

a. Nematodes

b. Cestodes

c. Acanthocephala

d. Protozoa

77. **The Casoni test is used for the diagnosis of:**

a. Hydatiosis

b. Taeniasis

c. Dipylidiosis

d. Monieziosis

78. **Seizures, intracranial hypertension, depression and psychosis are caused by infection with:**

a. *Taenia solium*

b. *Taenia saginata*

c. *Taenia serialis*

d. *Taenia hydatigena*

79. **A rectal swab should be taken for the diagnosis of:**

a. *Taenia saginata*

b. *Hymenolepis nana*

c. a and b

d. *Taenia solium*

80. **Neotropical echinococcosis is caused by which cestode?**

a. *Echinococcus multilocularis*

b. *Echinococcus oligarthus*

c. *Echinococcus vogeli*

d. None of these

81. **The recombinant vaccine Cysvax is designed for prevention of:**

   a. *Taenia solium*

   b. *Taenia saginata*

   c. *Taenia serialis*

   d. *Taenia hydatigena*

82. **The tapeworm affecting subcutaneous tissue of dog is:**

   a. *Taenia multiceps*

   b. *Oestrus ovis* larvae

   c. *Taenia serialis*

   d. *Taenia hydatigena*

83. **The *Cysticercus bovis* form of *Taenia saginata* in animals causes:**

   a. Measly pork

   b. Measly beef

   c. Butcher's jelly

   d. All of these

84. **Nodule formation in the intestine of poultry occurs due to:**

   a. *Railletina ecchinobothrida*

   b. *R. tetragona*

   c. *Raillletina cesticellus*

   d. All of these

85. **The most pathogenic tapeworm of poultry is:**

   a. *Railletina ecchinobothrida*

   b. *R. tetragona*

   c. *Raillletina cesticellus*

   d. *Davainea proglottina*

86. **Square-shaped eggs with a well-developed pyriform apparatus, measuring up to 75 mm in length are seen in:**

    a. *M. benedeni*

    b. *M. expansa*

    c. *Anoplocephala perfoliata*

    d. None of these

87. **What causes the deposition of black fluke pigment in small ruminants?**

    a. *Fasciola hepatica*

    b. *Fasciola gignatica*

    c. *Fascioloides magna*

    d. *Fasciolopsis buski*

88. **Which trematode is responsible for lizard poisoning in cats?**

    a. *Platynosum fastosum*

    b. *Fascoloides magna*

    c. *Eurythelminthes squamula*

    d. *Nanophytes salmonicola*

89. **In dogs, what does a history of chronic, deep, intermittent cough, combined with a diet of crab or crayfish suggest the presence of?**

    a. *Paragonimus westernmani*

    b. *Prosthogonimus ovatus*

    c. *Schistosoma haematobium*

    d. *Nanophytes samonicola*

90. **The Schistosoma species found in the messentaric vein of dogs**

    a. *Austrobilharzia* spp.

    b. *Heterobilharzia Americanum*

    c. *Schistosoma spindale*

    d. *Schistosoma nasale*

91. **Flukes found in the pancreatic duct of racoons and foxes indicate the presence of:**

    a. *Eurytrema procyonis*

    b. *Eurytrema pancreaticum*

    c. *Clonorchis sinensis*

    d. All of these

92. **The correct dose rate of praziquantel for treatment of schistosomosis in cattle is:**

    a. 10 mg/kg BWT

    b. 15 mg/kg BWT

    c. 30 mg/kg BWT

    d. 50 mg/kg BWT

93. **Flukes causing cholangiocarcinoma include:**

    a. *Opisthorchis viverrni*

    b. *Chlonorchis sinensis*

    c. *Eurytrema pancreaticum*

    d. a and b

94. **Impaired egg-laying, soft eggs, eggs with no shells at all, or amorphous masses full of flukes are indicative of:**

    a. *Paragonimus westernmani*

    b. *Prosthognimus ovatus*

    c. *Eurytrema pancreaticum*

    d. All of these

95. **Frank haemorrhagic duodenitis, severe enteritis, possible necrosis and haemorrhage in cattle and buffalo are characteristic signs of:**

    a. Schistosomosis

    b. Paramphistomosis

    c. Fasciolosis

    d. Paragonimiasis

96. **Pale mucous membrane, depraved appetite, submandibular swelling and loss of weight in elephants are suggestive of:**

    a. *Fasciola hepatica*

    b. *Fascola giantica*

    c. *Fasciola jacksoni*

    d. *Fscioloides magna*

97. **The drug of choice for treatment of liver fluke infection in Asian elephants is:**

    a. Nitroxynil

    b. Praziquantel

    c. Oxyclozanide

    d. All of these

98. **A cauliflower-like growth in the nasal mucosa is indicative of:**

    a. *Schistosoma spindale*

    b. *Schistosoma nasale*

    c. *Schistosoma haematobium*

    d. *Schistosoma bovis*

99. **The drug of choice for nasal schistomosis in buffalo is:**

    a. Lithium antibody thiomalate

    b. Fendendazole

    c. Oxycloazanide

    d. All of these

100. **Which type of *Fasciola* spp. causes intestinal disorder characterized by diarrhoea, abdominal pain, fever, ascites and intestinal obstruction in humans?**

    a. *Fasciola hepatica*

    b. *Fasciola gigantica*

    c. *Fasciolopsis buski*

    d. *Fascioloides magna*

101. The McLean County System of swine sanitization is followed for controlling which nematode?

a. *Ascaris suum*

b. *Haemonchus contortus*

c. *Trichostrongylus axei*

d. *Stephaneurus dentatus*

102. A 'rat-tailed' appearance in horses is associated with:

a. *Strongylus equi*

b. *Oxyuris equi*

c. *Parascaris equorum*

d. *Strongylus edentatus*

103. Diarrhoea, steatorrhea (fat in faeces), colic and passing mud-coloured, evil-smelling faeces in cattle/buffalo are characteristic of:

a. *Toxocara vitulorum*

b. *Oxyuris equi*

c. *Parascaris equorum*

d. *Strongylus equi*

104. What is the name for arrow-headed roundworm in dogs?

a. *Toxocara canis*

b. *Toxocara vitulorum*

c. *Toxascaris leonina*

d. *Ascaris suum*

105. The drug of choice for Ascarid infection is:

a. Piperazine

b. Albendazole

c. Praziquantel

d. Triclabendazole

106. Which ascarid worm has an indirect lifecycle?

a. *Parascaris equorum*

b. *Oxyuris equi*

c. *Toxocara canis*

d. *Subulura brumpti*

107. Instead of faecal examination, perineal swab is taken for the diagnosis of:

a. *Parascaris equorum*

b. *Oxyuris equi*

c. *Toxocara canis*

d. *Toxocara vitulorum*

108. Foals 3 to 9 months of age are commonly affected with which nematode?

a. *Parascaris equorum*

b. *Oxyuris equi*

c. *Strongylus equinus*

d. *Toxocara vitulorum*

109. Which method of faecal examination is used for the diagnosis of nematodal infection?

a. Direct

b. Gross

c. Floatation

d. Sedimentation

110. Autoinfection is caused by which ascarid worm?

a. *Enterobius vermicularis*

b. *Oxyuris equi*

c. *Toxocara canis*

d. *Toxocara vitulorum*

111. **Vitamin A, B and B12 deficiency occurs as a result of which infection?**

    a. *Heterakis gallinarum*

    b. *Ascaridia galli*

    c. *Subulura brumpti*

    d. All of these

112. **Black head or entero-hepatitis in turkeys is transmitted by which nematode?**

    a. *Heterakis gallinarum*

    b. *Ascaridia galli*

    c. *Subulura brumpti*

    d. All of these

113. **Visceral larva migrans in young children up to 5 years of age occurs due to which infection?**

    a. *Parascaris equorum*

    b. *Oxyuris equi*

    c. *Toxocara canis*

    d. *Toxocara vitulorum*

114. **Calves must be dewormed within 10 to 15 days of birth to prevent infection with what?**

    a. *Parascaris equorum*

    b. *Oxyuris equi*

    c. *Toxocara canis*

    d. *Toxocara vitulorum*

115. **Varying degrees of fibrosis in the liver in the form of 'milk spot' is associated with:**

    a. *Parascaris equorum*

    b. *Oxyuris equi*

    c. *Toxocara canis*

    d. *Ascaris suum*

116. **About two lakhs eggs per day are laid by which female ascarid worm?**

    a. *Ascaris suum*

    b. *Oxyuris equi*

    c. *Toxocara canis*

    d. *Toxocara vitulorum*

117. **Which nematode has an hour-glass shaped oesophagus?**

    a. *Ascaris suum*

    b. *Oxyuris equi*

    c. *Toxocara canis*

    d. *Toxocara vitulorum*

118. **'Bursate nematodes' belong to the order:**

    a. Ascaridida

    b. Strongylida

    c. Spirurida

    d. Rhabditida

119. **Endarteritis and thrombus formation in the cranial artery in equines occurs due to which nematode?**

    a. *S. vulgaris*

    b. *S. edentatus*

    c. *S. equinus*

    d. None of these

120. **Which nematode, with a slightly inflated cephalic vesicle, occurs in the colon of sheep, goats, cattle and other ruminants?**

    a. *S. vulgaris*

    b. *S. edentatus*

    c. *S. equinus*

    d. *Chabertia ovina*

121. The nodular worm with a cone-shaped mouth collar that occurs in sheep and goats is:

a. *Oesophagostomum columbianum*

b. *Oesophagostomum radiatum*

c. *Oesophagostomum venulosum*

d. *O. dentatum*

122. What is the likely cause of young chickens suffering from dyspnoea, asphyxia, shaking and tossing of the head, along with coughing and gaping?

a. *Heterakis gallinarum*

b. *Ascaridia galli*

c. *Subulura brumpti*

d. *Syngamus trachea*

123. What is the kidney worm in swine called?

a. *Stephaneurus dentatus*

b. *Ascaris suum*

c. *O. dentatum*

d. *Dioctophyma renale*

124. Which hookworm is found in cats?

a. *Ancylostoma caninum*

b. *A. braziliense*

c. *A. tubaeformae*

d. *A. duodenale*

125. Oedema in the intermandibular region (bottle jaw) can be the result of infection with:

a. *Bunostomum trignocephalum*

b. *Haemonchus contortus*

c. a and b

d. *Ostertagia ostertagi*

126. **In calves, gastric mucosa causing raised, plaque-like lesions with sharply demarcated borders, similar to ringworm lesions, result from:**

    a. *Trichostrongylus axei*

    b. *Haemonchus contortus*

    c. *Ostertagia ostertagi*

    d. *Cooperia punctata*

127. **How are hookworm and strongyloides infection usually acquired?**

    a. Bite of the adult

    b. Ingestion of contaminated food

    c. Contact of skin with infected soil

    d. None of these

128. **What is the causative agent of Cochin China diarrhoea?**

    a. *Ancylostoma duodenale*

    b. *Strongyloides stercoralis*

    c. *Capillaria philipinensis*

    d. *Necator americanus*

129. **Mango fly is the vector for what?**

    a. *Onchocerca volvulous*

    b. Loa loa

    c. *Onchocerca gibsoni*

    d. All of these

130. **Which parasite does not result in human infection passed on by pigs and dogs?**

    a. *Ecchinoccoccus granulosus*

    b. *Trichinella spiralis*

    c. *Ascaris lumbricoides*

    d. *Taenia solium*

131. **Which of the following statements concerning hookworm infection is incorrect?**

    a. Hookworm causes anaemia

    b. Hookworm can be diagnosed by finding trophozoite in the stool

    c. Infection is acquired by humans when filariform larvae penetrate the skin

    d. Hookworm infection is caused by *Necator americanus*

132. **Each of the following parasites passes through the lungs during the course of human infection with the exception of:**

    a. *Necator americanus*

    b. *Wucheria bancrofti*

    c. *Ascaris lumbricoides*

    d. *Taenia solium*

133. **Rectal prolapse can occur as a result of which nematodal infection?**

    a. *Enterobius vermicularis*

    b. *Oxyuris equi*

    c. *Trichuris trichuria*

    d. *Capillaria philipinensis*

134. **Parthenogenesis occurs in which worm?**

    a. Ascaris

    b. Enterobius

    c. Hookworm

    d. Strongyoides

135. **Ground itch occurs as part of which worm infection?**

    a. Toxocara

    b. Enterobius

    c. Ascaris

    d. Hookworm

136. **The Graham's test is used for which diagnosis?**

a. Toxocara

b. Ascaris

c. Trichinella

d. Enterobius

137. **How many times do Strongyloides L1 larvae have to moult in order to enter a free-living cycle?**

a. Once

b. Twice

c. 3 times

d. 4 times

138. **Which 4 worms have lifecycles involving migration to the lungs, being coughed up, swallowed and then travelling down to the intestine?**

a. Strongyloides, hookworm, ascaris and paragonimus

b. Trichuris, hookworm, strongyloides and ascaris

c. Taenia, dicrocoelium, hookworm and enterobius

d. Schistosoma, opisthorchis, ascaris and dipylidium

139. **Loeffler's syndrome occurs in which nematode infection?**

a. *Trichuri trichuria*

b. *Ascaris lumbricoides*

c. *Capillaria philippinensis*

d. *Enterobius vermicularis*

140. **Which larvae can usually be found in fresh faeces?**

a. Taenia

b. Hookworm

c. Strongyloides

d. Enterobius

141. **Catarrhal gastritis with a large amount of mucus and ulceration to the stomach mucosa is characteristic of:**

   a. *Habronema muscae*

   b. *Habronema majus*

   c. *Draschia megastoma*

   d. All of these

142. **Nodule formation resembling tumour in the stomach mucosa is a characteristic of:**

   a. *Habronema muscae*

   b. *H. majus*

   c. *Draschia megastoma*

   d. All of these

143. **In horses, *Draschia megastoma* causes what?**

   a. Summer sore

   b. Bursati

   c. Granular conjunctivitis

   d. All of these

144. **Which eye worm may be found in the nictitating membrane of dogs?**

   a. *Thelazia rhodesi*

   b. *Thelazia lacrymalis*

   c. *Thelazia callipeda*

   d. *Setaria digitata*

145. **The nematode responsible for tumours in the oesophagus is:**

   a. *Spirocerca lupi*

   b. *Thelazia lacrymalis*

   c. *Thelazia callipeda*

   d. *Setaria digitata*

146. **The nematode present in the nictitating membrane of birds is likely to be:**

    a. *Spirocerca lupi*

    b. *Oxyspirura mansoni*

    c. *Thelazia callipeda*

    d. *Setaria digitata*

147. **Which nematode, showing sexual dimorphism, may be present in the proventriculus and gizzard of poultry?**

    a. *Tetrameres mohtedai*

    b. *Oxyspirura mansoni*

    c. *Thelazia callipeda*

    d. *Setaria digitata*

148. **Which nematode lies in a zig-zag fashion and is found embedded in the oesophageal mucosa?**

    a. *Spirocerca lupi*

    b. *Oxyspirura mansoni*

    c. *Gongylonema pulchrum*

    d. *Setaria digitata*

149. **Which nematode is responsible for VLM, CLM and OLM in man?**

    a. *Toxocara canis*

    b. *Ancylostoma caninum*

    c. *Ganthostoma spinigerum*

    d. *Gongylonema pulchrum*

150. **Congestive heart failure, liver failure syndrome and peripheral oedema in dogs indicates the presence of:**

    a. *Setaria digitata*

    b. *Dirofilaria immitis*

    c. *Dipetalonema reconditum*

    d. All of these

151.   **What is swollen belly syndrome in children caused by?**

    a. *Strongyloides papillosus*

    b. *Strongyloides fuelleborni*

    c. *Strongyloides stercoralis*

    d. *Strongyloides mirabilis*

152.   **The adulticide used for treatment of canine heartworm disease is known as what?**

    a. Thiacetarsamide

    b. Melarsoprol

    c. a and b

    d. Dithiazine iodide

153.   **Which drugs are used to prevent heartworm disease?**

    a. DEC

    b. Mebendazole

    c. Ivermectin and milbemycin

    d. All of these

154.   **Which microfilariacide is used to treat canine heartworm disease?**

    a. Dithiazine iodide

    b. Levamisole

    c. Avermectin B1a

    d. All of these

155.   **Strongyloides papillosus is commonly known as:**

    a. Stomach worm

    b. Oesophageal worm

    c. Thread worm

    d. Lung worm

156. **Which nematode causes foot rot associated with *Bacteriodes nodosus*?**

   a. *Strongyloides papillosus*

   b. *Strongyloides stercoralis*

   c. *Strongyloides mirabilis*

   d. All of these

157. **A homogenic and heterogenic life cycle is seen in:**

   a. *Strongylus vulgaris*

   b. *Draschia megastoma*

   c. *Strongyloides papillosus*

   d. All of these

158. **'Worm nest' or nodule formation in cattle and buffalo is caused by:**

   a. *Onchocerca volvulous*

   b. *Onchocerca gibsoni*

   c. *Onchocerca gutterosa*

   d. *Onchocerca cervicalis*

159. **Which filarial nematode, transmitted by *Mansonia* spp. and anopheles mosquito, is present in the lymphatic system of primates and carnivores?**

   a. *Loa loa*

   b. *Dirofilaria repens*

   c. *Brugia malayi*

   d. *Wucheria bancrofti*

160. **In horses, the nematode *Onchocerca cervicalis* causes what?**

   a. Worm nest

   b. Mazzoti reaction

   c. Poll evil

   d. Lameness

161. **Elephantitis in humans is caused by which nematode?**

    a. *Loa loa*

    b. *Dirofilaria repens*

    c. *Brugia malayi*

    d. *Wucheria bancrofti*

162. **Which filarial nematode causes river blindness/periodic opthalmia?**

    a. *Onchocerca volvulous*

    b. *Onchocerca gibsoni*

    c. *Onchocerca gutterosa*

    d. *Onchocerca cervicalis*

163. **Which filarial nematode residing in the subcutaneous and intermuscular connective tissue of cattle and buffalo forms haemorrhagic nodules and bleeding points after 242–319 days of infection, finally leading to summer bleeding/haemorrhagic dermatitis?**

    a. *Parafilaria bovicola*

    b. *Dirofilaria repens*

    c. *Brugia malayi*

    d. *P. multipapillosa*

164. **The Mazzoti reaction is seen with which anthelmintic?**

    a. Ivermectin

    b. Milbemycin

    c. Diethyl carbamazine

    d. All of these

165. **'Crisis phenomenon' is seen in:**

    a. *Toxocara canis*

    b. *Ancylostoma caninum*

    c. *Bunostomum trignocephalum*

    d. *Gnathostoma spinigerum*

166. **'Self-cure phenomenon' in sheep is mainly due to:**

    a. *Moniezia expansa*

    b. *Haemonchus controtus*

    c. *Ostertagia ostertagi*

    d. *Paracooperia* spp.

167. **Dictol vaccine for cattle and buffalo is produced for the prevention of:**

    a. *Dictyocaulus viviparous*

    b. *Dictyocaulus filarial*

    c. *Dictyocaulus arnfieldi*

    d. *Metastrongylus apri*

168. **Which anthelmintic drug is used to treat hump sore in cattle?**

    a. Albendazole

    b. Milbemycin

    c. Fenbendazole

    d. Ivermectin

169. **Babervax vaccine is designed to prevent:**

    a. *Moniezia expansa*

    b. *Haemonchus controtus*

    c. *Ostertagia ostertagi*

    d. *Oesophagostomum columbianum*

170. **Ancylol vaccine is administered against:**

    a. *Toxocara canis*

    b. *Dirofilaria immitis*

    c. *Ancylostoma caninum*

    d. *Toxascaris leonina*

171. **The Baemann technique is used to produce cultures of which nematode?**

    a. *Paragonimum westermani*

    b. *Dirofilaria immitis*

    c. *Dictyocaulus viviparous*

    d. *Haemonchus contortus*

172. **Knott's technique is used to detect:**

    a. Stomach worm

    b. Filarial worm

    c. Blood fluke

    d. Lung worm

173. **Haemono melasma ilei is caused by:**

    a. *Strongyloides papillosus*

    b. *Strongylus edentates*

    c. *Strongyloides mirabilis*

    d. *Strongylus vulgaris*

174. **A FAMCHA chart is used to diagnose anaemia associated with:**

    a. *Moniezia expansa*

    b. *Haemonchus controtus*

    c. *Ostertagia ostertagi*

    d. *Oesophagostomum columbianum*

175. **Trichinellosis is acquired from:**

    a. Contaminated water

    b. Contaminated soil

    c. Ingestion of bear or pork meat

    d. All of these

176. **A bentonite floculaton test is used to diagnose:**

    a. Trichinosis

    b. Trichellosis

    c. Haemonchosis

    d. Cappilllariosis

177. **Which acanthocephalan nematode in dogs and cats causes rabiform signs in infected animals?**

    a. *Mecracanthorhyncus* spp.

    b. *Trichuris* spp.

    c. *Oncicola canis*

    d. *Diphyllobothrium latum*

178. **Helminth therapy for autoimmune disease primarily uses:**

    a. *Trichuris suis*

    b. *Necator americanus*

    c. *Trichuris trichuria*

    d. All of these

179. **Which drug is effective against cestode?**

    a. Praziquantel

    b. Ivermectin

    c. Pyrantal pamoate

    d. Albendazole

180. **The nematode responsible for parasitic otitis is:**

    a. *Rhabditis ovis*

    b. *Spirocerca lupi*

    c. *Cooperia punctata*

    d. *Nematodirus* spp.

181. **A 'Morocco leather'-like appearance of the skin is due to infection with:**

   a. *Ostertagia osteratagi*

   b. *Spirocerca lupi*

   c. *Cooperia punctate*

   d. *Nematodirus* spp.

182. **Balliup in horses is due to:**

   a. *Parascaris equorum*

   b. *Strongylus vulgaris*

   c. *Oxyuris equi*

   d. *Strongylus edentatus*

183. **In cattle and buffalo, hump sores occur due to:**

   a. *Stephanofilaria assamensis*

   b. *Stephanofilaria zaheri*

   c. *Dioctophyma renale*

   d. *Angiostrongylus cantonensis*

184. **Haemorrhagic warts in tracheal bifurcation in dogs occur due to:**

   a. *Filaroides osleri*

   b. *Toxocara canis*

   c. *Dioctophyma renale*

   d. *Angiostrongylus cantonensis*

185. **In horses, verminous aneurysm in the cranial messentaric artery occurs due to:**

   a. *Strongylus vulgaris*

   b. *Strongyloides papillosu*

   c. *Strongylus edentates*

   d. All of these

186. **Protein-losing gastropathy in horses is associated with what?**

    a. *Trichostrongylus* spp.

    b. *Nematodirus* spp.

    c. *Strongylus vulgaris*

    d. a and b

187. **Overdosing with which anthelmintic can lead to severe toxicity in animals?**

    a. Ivermectin

    b. Levamisole

    c. Fenbendazole

    d. Praziquantel

188. **An anthelmintic should not be used haphazardly to maintain which population of parasite?**

    a. Resistant

    b. Dominant

    c. Refugia

    d. Recessive

189. **The anthelmintic contraindicated in pregnancy is:**

    a. Fenbendazole

    d. Piperazine

    c. Albendazole

    d. Praziquantel

190. ***Angiostrongylus cantonensis* in rats causes:**

    a. Eosinophilic meningitis

    b. Basophilic meningitis

    c. a and b

    d. None of these

191. **Young puppies below 1 year old and smaller breeds of dog are predisposed to:**
    a. Ancylostomosis
    b. Toxocarosis
    c. Gnathostomosis
    d. All of these

192. **Pale mucous membrane, diarrhoea with bloody mucous and passing tarry red-coloured faeces in dogs is characteristic of:**
    a. Ancylostomosis
    b. Toxocarosis
    c. Gnathostomosis
    d. All of these

193. **Anal dragging in dogs is caused by:**
    a. Dipylidosis
    b. Ancylostomosis
    c. Diphyllobothriosis
    d. All of these

194. **A periparturient egg rise in nematodes occurs due to which hormone?**
    a. Oesotrogen
    b. Progesterone
    c. Prolactin
    d. Lutenizing hormone

195. **Parasitic bronchitis or 'husk hoose' in cattle occurs mainly due to:**
    a. *Dioctophyma renale*
    b. *Dictyocaulus viviparous*
    c. *Dictyocaulus arnfieldi*
    d. *Dictyocaulus filaria*

196.   The following helminth can cause right kidney damage in dogs, including blockage, hydronephrosis, and renal parenchyma destruction:

a. *Dioctophyma renale*

b. *Stephaneurus dentatus*

c. *Metastrongylus apri*

d. All of these

197.   In mule deer and black-tailed deer, *Elaeophora schneideri* causes:

a. Filarial dermatosis

b. Clear-eyed blindness

c. Sorehead

d. All of these

198.   The ascarid worm found in the small intestine of raccoons is:

a. *Ascaris suum*

b. *Capillaria hepatica*

c. *Baylisascaris procyonis*

d. None of these

199.   Rear leg paresis, ataxia, circling, inability to stand, cervical scoliosis and blindness occur in an accidental host (e.g. moose, elk, sheep, goats, antelope and alpaca) due to:

a. *Parlephostrongylus tenius*

b. *Baylisascaris procyonis*

c. *Setaria cervi*

d. *Elaeophora schneideri*

200.   The first line of defence for helminthic infection is:

a. Monocyte

b. Neutrophil

c. Eosinophil

d. Lymphocyte

Answers

1.	a	**31.**	c	**61.**	c	**91.**	a
2.	c	**32.**	c	**62.**	b	**92.**	c
3.	b	**33.**	a	**63.**	d	**93.**	d
4.	b	**34.**	a	**64.**	a	**94.**	b
5.	c	**35.**	d	**65.**	d	**95.**	b
6.	c	**36.**	d	**66.**	a	**96.**	c
7.	b	**37.**	a	**67.**	b	**97.**	a
8.	d	**38.**	b	**68.**	c	**98.**	b
9.	b	**39.**	b	**69.**	a	**99.**	a
10.	d	**40.**	a	**70.**	a	**100.**	c
11.	c	**41.**	b	**71.**	c	**101.**	a
12.	c	**42.**	a	**72.**	c	**102.**	b
13.	d	**43.**	b	**73.**	d	**103.**	a
14.	b	**44.**	c	**74.**	b	**104.**	a
15.	c	**45.**	a	**75.**	d	**105.**	a
16.	d	**46.**	c	**76.**	b	**106.**	d
17.	d	**47.**	b	**77.**	a	**107.**	b
18.	b	**48.**	c	**78.**	a	**108.**	a
19.	c	**49.**	a	**79.**	c	**109.**	c
20.	c	**50.**	c	**80.**	b	**110.**	a
21.	a	**51.**	a	**81.**	a	**111.**	b
22.	c	**52.**	b	**82.**	c	**112.**	a
23.	c	**53.**	b	**83.**	b	**113.**	c
24.	d	**54.**	c	**84.**	a	**114.**	d
25.	c	**55.**	d	**85.**	a	**115.**	d
26.	b	**56.**	c	**86.**	d	**116.**	a
27.	d	**57.**	d	**87.**	a	**117.**	b
28.	d	**58.**	c	**88.**	c	**118.**	b
29.	c	**59.**	d	**89.**	a	**119.**	a
30.	a	**60.**	c	**90.**	b	**120.**	d

(Continued)

121.	a	141.	a	161.	d	181.	a
122.	d	142.	b	162.	a	182.	a
123.	a	143.	d	163.	a	183.	a
124.	c	144.	c	164.	c	184.	a
125.	c	145.	a	165.	b	185.	a
126.	a	146.	b	166.	b	186.	d
127.	c	147.	a	167.	a	187.	a
128.	b	148.	c	168.	d	188.	c
129.	b	149.	c	169.	d	189.	c
130.	c	150.	b	170.	c	190.	a
131.	b	151.	b	171.	c	191.	a
132.	b	152.	c	172.	b	192.	a
133.	c	153.	d	173.	b	193.	a
134.	d	154.	d	174.	b	194.	c
135.	d	155.	d	175.	c	195.	b
136.	d	156.	a	176.	b	196.	a
137.	d	157.	c	177.	c	197.	d
138.	d	158.	b	178.	d	198.	c
139.	b	159.	c	179.	b	199.	a
140.	c	160.	c	180.	a	200.	c

www.ingramcontent.com/pod-product-compliance
Lightning Source LLC
Chambersburg PA
CBHW050803270326
41926CB00025B/4524